# Stretching Exercises For Seniors

Simple Movements to Improve Posture, Decrease Back Pain, and Prevent Injury After 60

**Baz Thompson**

© Copyright 2021 - All Rights Reserved.

The content contained within this book may not be reproduced, duplicated or transmitted without direct written permission from the author or the publisher.

Under no circumstances will any blame or legal responsibility be held against the publisher, or author, for any damages, reparation, or monetary loss due to the information contained within this book, either directly or indirectly.

## Legal Notice:

This book is copyright protected. It is only for personal use. You cannot amend, distribute, sell, use, quote or paraphrase any part, or the content within this book, without the consent of the author or publisher.

## Disclaimer Notice:

Please note the information contained within this document is for educational and entertainment purposes only. All effort has been executed to present accurate, up to date, reliable, complete information. No warranties of any kind are declared or implied. Readers acknowledge that the author is not engaged in the rendering of legal, financial, medical or professional advice. The content within this book has been derived from various sources. Please consult a licensed professional before attempting any techniques outlined in this book.

By reading this document, the reader agrees that under no circumstances is the author responsible for any losses, direct or indirect, that are incurred as a result of the use of the information contained within this document, including, but not limited to, errors, omissions, or inaccuracies.

# Table of Contents

Introduction _____ 7

## Chapter 1: The Power Of Stretching

Our Bodies As We Age _____ 11
The Benefits of Stretching _____ 13
The Types of Stretching _____ 13
When, Where, and How to Stretch _____ 14
    When to Stretch _____ 15
    Where to Stretch _____ 16
    How to Stretch _____ 16

## Chapter 2: Morning Stretches

**Upper Body Stretches**

Overhead Stretch _____ 22
Cactus Arms _____ 23
Neck Roll Stretch _____ 24
Seated Spinal Twist _____ 25
Cat and Cow _____ 26

**Lower Body Stretches**

Seated Forward Bend _____ 28
Foot Point and Flex _____ 29
Half Kneeling Hip Flexor Stretch _____ 30
Lying Knees to Chest _____ 31
All Fours Side Bend _____ 32

## Chapter 3: Evening and Bedtime Stretches

### Upper Body Stretches

Bear Hug _____ 36
Seated Overhead Side Stretch _____ 37
Thread the Needle _____ 38
Floor Angels _____ 39
Child's Pose _____ 40

### Lower Body Stretches

Banana Stretch _____ 42
Windshield Wipers Stretch _____ 43
Reclined Figure Four _____ 44
Lying Spinal Twist _____ 45
Reclined Butterfly _____ 46

## Chapter 4: Pre-Activity Stretches

### Upper Body Stretches

Cross Body Shoulder Stretch _____ 50
Overhead Tricep Stretch _____ 51
Ear to Shoulder Neck Stretch _____ 52
Standing Chest Stretch _____ 53
Standing Torso Twist _____ 54

### Lower Body Stretches

Hurdler Hamstring Stretch _____ 56
Standing Calf Stretch _____ 57
Quad Stretch _____ 58
Seated Butterfly _____ 59
Standing Lunge _____ 60

## Chapter 5: Post-Activity Stretches

### Upper Body Stretches

Wrist Rotation Bicep Stretch _____ 64

Shoulder Rolls ........................................................................... 65
Eagle Arms Pose ....................................................................... 66
Superman Stretch .................................................................... 67
Lying Pectoral Stretch .............................................................. 68

### Lower Body Stretches

Lying Hamstring Stretch .......................................................... 70
Bridge Pose ............................................................................... 71
Happy Baby .............................................................................. 72
Square Pose .............................................................................. 73
Knee to Opposite Shoulder IT Band Stretch ........................... 74

## Chapter 6: Target Area Stretches

### Upper Body Stretches

Hand and Finger Tendon Glide ................................................ 78
Wrist Flexor and Extensor Stretch ........................................... 79
Wrist Ulnar and Radial Stretch ................................................ 80
Butterfly Wings Upper Back Stretch ....................................... 81
Cobra Abs ................................................................................. 82

### Lower Body Stretches

Toe Raises, Points, and Curls .................................................. 84
Toe Extension or Foot Flex ...................................................... 85
Ankle Alphabet ........................................................................ 86
Kneeling Shin Stretch .............................................................. 87
Hip Rotations ........................................................................... 88

## Conclusion ........................................................................... 89

## References ........................................................................... 91

# BEFORE YOU START READING

As a special gift, I included a logbook and a cookbook with a variety of recipes to suit all tastes and lifestyles and the best part is, you get access to all of them for free.

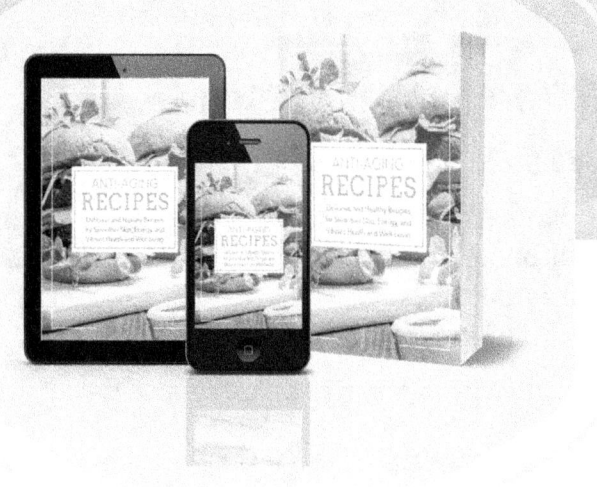

## What's in it for me?

- This cookbook is designed to strengthen your immune system, increase your energy and keep you feeling healthy well into your golden years.
- Recipes to help ensure that the aging process will be gentle and healthful.
- Workout Logbook to help you keep track of your accomplishments and progress. Log your progress to give you the edge you need to accomplish your goals.

# Introduction

Stretching is an activity you may think you don't need to do. You might say, "I'm not a gymnast or a football player. Why would I need to stretch?" While athletes of all kinds do practice stretching as part of their quest to maintain their competitive edge, all types of folks also stretch to benefit their bodies and general well-being. Regular stretching helps keep our muscles strong and pliable. This helps with flexibility in our muscles, ligaments, tendons, and joints (Harvard Health Publishing, 2013). By sustaining our flexibility, we keep our full range of motion, which allows us to continue the activities we enjoy.

Our normal range of activities that we do every day contributes to our need for stretching. When we stay seated for any length of time, the muscles in the back of our legs become tight. This makes it difficult to straighten our legs all the way, resulting in an increase in pain when we walk. Something as simple as walking can become harder to do when our muscles are tight and joints are stiff. When we ask our tight muscles to suddenly spring into action, for something fun like dancing with our partner or for something imperative like jumping out of the way of an oncoming bicycle, they may pull or tear because of the strain. Muscles that are not strong enough to support us in everyday tasks can lead to falls and other serious injuries.

Regular stretching keeps our muscles from contraction and stiffness. By keeping them elongated, flexible, and healthy, we protect our joints, ligaments, and tendons as well. It is not necessary to stretch all our muscles every day. Doctors and physical therapists like David Nolan of Massachusetts General Hospital recommend concentrating most stretches on the major muscle groups that affect our mobility (Harvard Health Publishing, 2013). This includes lower body muscles such as hip flexors, hamstrings (back of thigh), quadriceps (front of thigh), and calves. Also recommended are upper body stretches that target areas of tension like the neck, shoulders, and lower back.

We've all heard the saying that Rome was not built in a day, and the same can be said for flexibility. Stretching a few times will not make you less stiff and more flexible. The effects of stretching are cumulative, meaning that they build over time. Just as your stiffness and immobility did not happen overnight, the looseness and limberness of your muscles will not happen right away. It can take months to become more flexible and it takes regular stretching to maintain it. The result is strong, supple muscles that are flexible and supportive of joints and connective tissue. This contributes to our quality of life, especially as we age.

This book looks at stretching as a way to maintain good posture, decrease back pain, and help prevent injury as we progress past the age of sixty. The older population can especially benefit from a regular stretching routine. Getting older can sometimes mean a decrease in strenuous activity, an increase in surgeries, and less mobility because of disease or age. While stretching can't fix everything, it can bring movement and increased flexibility back to a person's life in their older years. In the first chapter, we will look at what happens to our bodies as we get older and the particular benefits that come from regular stretching. We will also learn about the types of stretching and when, where, and how to do it. The following chapters are dedicated to the times of day to stretch such as morning, evening, pre-activity, and post-activity. Included are the explanations and illustrations of each stretch and what areas of the body they benefit. Lastly, there is a chapter on target area stretches that focus on the smaller muscles of the body that profit from stretching.

As always, check with your doctor or healthcare provider before starting on any exercise or stretching regimen particularly if you have had a recent injury, are recovering from surgery, or have a chronic health condition.

Thank you so much for downloading my book. I would love to hear your thoughts so be sure to leave a review on Amazon. This will help many other people who are in the same situation as you find my book. It would mean a lot to me.

## Scan the QR code to leave a review

Are you ready? Let's get your fitness education and training started!

# The Power of Stretching

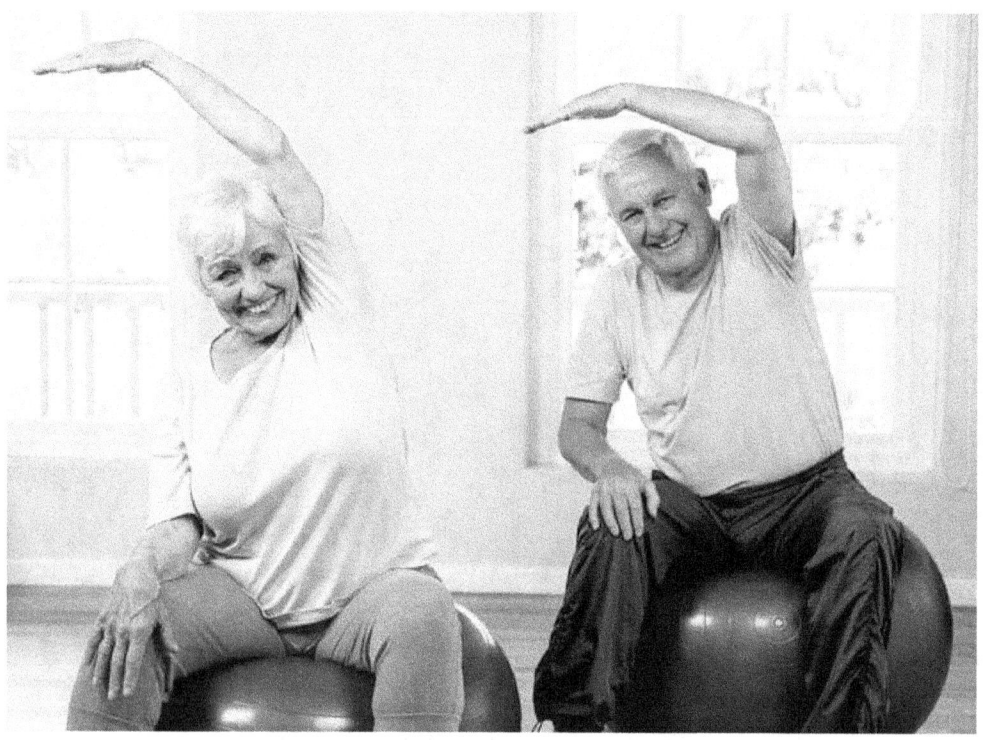

Stretching is good for our bodies at any age, but in this chapter, we will examine why it is especially important to stretch as we get older. We will take a look at what happens physiologically to our bodies as we progress in years, including what things we can do to prevent ourselves from further problems and injury. Next, we will talk about the benefits of stretching and why even a little bit of daily stretching will keep us from pain and stiffness. We will learn about the types of stretches we can do that are beneficial, plus highlight what kinds of stretches to avoid. Finally, we will talk about when, where, and how to stretch for everyone from beginner to experienced stretchers.

## Our Bodies As We Age

In the past, the older population was lumped together in one large group known as the elderly. With average life spans increasing, however, older adults are now subdivided into smaller age range groups. The adult population over 65 can be divided into three groups:

- **Young Old (ages 65 to 74).**
- **Middle Old (ages 75 to 84).**
- **Old Old (ages 85 and older).**

Someone who is 65 years old will have very different muscle strength, cognitive awareness, physical abilities, and injury recovery time than someone who is 90 years old. In one study, it was found that those in the Young Old group had lower hospital admission rates and quicker hospital discharge rates than those in the Old Old group (Lee, et al., 2018). It is important to note that our chronological age, the actual number of years we have lived on earth, is only one way to measure our age. There is also our biological age to consider.

Biological age refers to our level of physical fitness, mental acuity, and overall health. We can see this when we compare two people who are the same chronological age but who differ greatly in their biological age. One person who is 70 years old may have arthritis, limited mobility in their hands and knees, constant brain fog, and consume a diet high in processed foods and sugar. The other 70 year old person may have diabetes but still have the ability to play tennis twice a week, practice yoga daily, complete crossword puzzles regularly, and eat lots of fresh vegetables and fruits. Chronological age is something we don't have control over, but our biological age is one that we exert some control by the choices we make.

Our level of physical and mental fitness, or biological age, has several contributing factors. One factor is the DNA that we are born with in our cells. Some people are born with a propensity for disease or frailty that is determined by their inherited genes. Obviously, this factor cannot be changed, regardless of what we do. There are other factors, however, that are in our control. These factors include healthy food choices; regular exercise and stretching; maintenance of mental sharpness, emotional balance, and social connections.

We know that as the years pass, we get older and our bodies change. With the advancement of medical technology and preventative medicine, humans are able to live longer and have a better quality of life than our ancestors. However, we cannot stop the natural decline of certain faculties and the damage that happens to our cells with the passage of time. When we are young, our cells have the ability to repair themselves quickly and with minimal draw from energy resources in the body (National Center for Biotechnology Information, U.S. Library of Medicine, 2020). As we get older, the cells do not turn over as quickly and that slow down in cell turnover adds up, eventually resulting in signs of aging.

Our bodies are composed of many different types of cells. Some cells are short-lived, so they are constantly being replaced by new ones. An example of this type of cell is our skin cells. As we grow older, this replacement doesn't happen as quickly. With skin cells, this slow down in replacement cells can be seen in the form of skin wrinkles, less elasticity, and dryness. Other cells are long-lived, but when they die they are never replaced. Cells in the brain are an example of this type.

Muscle cells, even in older adults, are self-renewing. One of the natural consequences of growing older is a loss of muscle mass and strength which contributes to frailty and immobility. This often results in falls and an increased risk for injury. Certain lifestyle choices, however, can help slow down the loss of muscle. According to a recent study (McCormick & Vasilaki, 2018), these factors include:

- **Increase in protein consumption.**
- **Aerobic exercise.**
- **Resistance training.**
- **Other forms of physical activity like stretching.**

Paying attention to these factors and choosing to apply them in our lives helps slow the loss of muscle mass and muscle strength as we grow older. Some researchers have concluded that "...Exercise training and proper nutrition can have dramatic effects on muscle mass and strength" (Volpi, et al., 2004).

# The Benefits of Stretching

When it is done correctly, stretching feels good. The American Council on Exercise says that flexibility is an essential part of fitness and should be incorporated into a regular workout program (American Council on Exercise, 2014). They list 10 benefits of stretching, including:

- Increased blood flow to muscles and joints, plus increased circulation of blood throughout the body.
- Loosening of muscles in preparation for exercise.
- Relieves post-exercise aches and pains.
- Improves range of motion and decreases muscle stiffness.
- Decreases resistance of muscles, leading to possible decrease in injury.
- Improves posture and alignment of shoulder, spine, and hip muscles.
- Allows muscle relaxation and reduces muscle tension.
- Reduces lower back pain.
- Creates more efficient joint movement which makes movements require less energy.
- Reduces overall stress in the body.

In a study done on women between the ages of 62 and 74, researchers looked specifically at the knee flexors of the women in the study. After three months of participating in an active stretching program, the women were found to have increased flexibility and torque (twisting ability) in their knee flexors, which are the muscles that surround and decrease the angle of the knees, such as the hamstrings (Batista, et al., 2009). This increase in flexibility provided more functional mobility in all the women.

# The Types of Stretching

When we think of stretching, we may remember how we used to stretch when we were in an elementary school physical education class. Do you remember standing and bending over, trying to touch your feet while bouncing from the waist? Or sitting on the floor, legs apart, and trying to touch your toes while stretching and bouncing? This type of stretching is known as ballistic stretching. The premise of ballistic stretching uses force, gravity, or momentum to stretch your muscle past its normal range of motion by repeatedly bouncing or pushing. While this mode of stretching has fallen out of favor because of the increased possibility of muscle tears and pulls, some professional athletes and dancers still use it. This type of stretching is not recommended for most people, and especially not for older adults.

Popular in today's medical and fitness worlds are dynamic stretching and static stretching. What is the difference between the two? Dynamic stretching is used prior to exercising, team sports, or any strenuous activity. The purpose of dynamic stretching is to get the muscles ready that you will be using in the activity by increasing the temperature of the muscles and decreasing any muscle stiffness. These stretches take your muscles and joints through the range of motion slowly before you perform them with more intensity and speed. Examples of dynamic stretches are walking lunges, torso twists, arm circles, and leg swings. Many dynamic stretches are sport specific, meaning they mimic the movement you will be doing in your particular sport or workout.

Static stretching is used after exercise to help you cool down and stretch out muscles, but it is also used as part of a routine stretching program to help maintain flexibility and mobility in your muscles and joints. Stretching a muscle as far as it can go without pain and holding the stretch for 30 to 60 seconds is the basic idea of static stretching. Holding a stretched position helps lengthen your muscles, increasing flexibility, and helps relax your muscles. Examples of static stretches are hamstring stretch, side bends, and hip flexor stretch. Static stretches are done standing, sitting, or lying down.

# When, Where, and How to Stretch

In this section, we will look at the basics of stretching and learn when, where, and how to stretch.

## When to Stretch

We have already touched on the importance of stretching before exercising or activity and afterwards. The pre-activity stretches are meant to warm up muscles for an increase in muscular activity through exercise, dance, or other sport. These stretches don't help with flexibility but are preparation for increased movement. Post-activity stretches are done while you are cooling down from an exercise or activity. Your muscles are easier to stretch because they are warm and supple, making them more flexible. But what about other times of the day that stretching can be done?

Stretching in the morning just after waking up is a great way to release tension and to help you gently wake up your body. The body heals and does repair work on itself while you are sleeping and that includes repair of muscles and other soft tissue (Walker, 2010). When you awaken in the morning, increasing your circulation flow brings blood and oxygen into your muscles at a higher rate and gets your body ready for the events of the day ahead. Morning stretches also help wake up your joints and alleviate any stiffness from them being still and immobile most of the night.

A short stretch break done several times during the day is helpful to keep joints and muscles loose and moving. If you do a lot of sitting for work or in your leisure time, it's important to get up and stretch your neck, upper back, lower back, and hips to keep them limber. Stretch breaks are also great ways to take a mental break from whatever work or activity you are doing. By concentrating on your body and the movements it is making as you stretch, along with some focused breathing, you can come back to your work relaxed and renewed.

Most people do not think of stretching in the evening before going to bed, but this is a great time to stretch! As we discussed earlier, your muscles and soft tissues like ligaments and tendons are repaired while you sleep. By stretching in the evening, you elongate and lengthen your muscles. This increased muscle length allows the repair and healing work to be done along the entire muscle (Walker, 2010). Also, stretching before bedtime is a way to wind down and relax. The slow, rhythmic movements of a gentle stretching routine, along with measured breathing, help signal the body and mind that sleep is coming.

## Where to Stretch

The best place to stretch is anywhere that you have enough room and are comfortable. This could be in your bedroom, living room, home gym, backyard, or garage. It is also possible to stretch outdoors at a park, beach, or open air sports facility. The important thing is to check the surroundings to be sure that you are stretching on a level surface to avoid any imbalances or falls. Having a padded exercise or yoga mat can be helpful, especially if you are doing stretches that involve kneeling, sitting, or lying on the ground. Seated stretches can be done from a chair at your desk, dining room table, or even in your car.

## How to Stretch

Stretching requires more than just bending over and reaching for your toes. Proper form such as breathing, variety, and alignment all contribute to getting the most out of your stretching routine. Being aware of common mistakes and avoiding them is also important.

Breathing seems like a natural thing to do. We all do it several thousand times a day. Proper breathing allows for full expansion of your entire lungs. Many people breathe by taking shallow breaths that cause their chest to rise and fall and their waist to contract and get small. These types of breaths miss filling the lower part of your lungs. The proper way to breathe, sometimes called belly breathing, is to breathe into your belly and diaphragm area. To do this, sit or lie down comfortably and breathe in through your nose. Your chest and belly should expand, and then exhale through your mouth. Belly breathing takes some practice, but gets easier as you practice it more.

Doing some stretching every day is a good idea, especially if you are working on flexibility or recovery of a particular muscle. Just as you wouldn't eat the same thing everyday or do the same exercise day in and day out, you also don't want to do the same stretches all the time. Including several different types of stretches is important to avoid any muscle imbalances or overworking of muscles.

Good posture and body alignment are important to avoid strain and injury, and that goes for stretching, too. Maintaining proper posture and good form as you stretch helps ensure that the muscles you are targeting are being stretched properly and that you are not putting unnecessary pressure on your neck or other joints. There is a tendency for some people to scrunch their shoulders or hunch over while stretching. This causes imbalance and undue tension on those areas that may lead to injury. Maintain good posture and alignment by keeping your back straight (but not rigid), shoulders down and away from your ears, and your jaw relaxed.

According to the Stretch Coach, author and stretching guru Brad Walker, there are some common mistakes that people make when they start out stretching (Walker, 2010). These include:

- Holding your breath. This causes muscles to tense up and become difficult to stretch. Breathe deeply using the belly breathing technique to relax muscles and increase circulation.
- Forgetting to warm up. Walker likens this to stretching old, dry rubber bands. They don't stretch very far and may snap. Take five minutes to warm up your muscles by walking in place to increase muscle temperature and make them more pliable.

- Stretching an injury. If injured, there should not be any stretching done for the first 72 hours. For the first two weeks, very gentle and light static stretching can be done. After that some dynamic stretching can slowly be reintroduced into your stretching routine.

- Stretching to the point of pain. When we stretch too hard, our muscles employ a built-in safety reflex. They naturally contract to get away and protect the body from the pain. Stretch only to where it is comfortable and a slight tension.

- Not holding the stretch long enough. Holding the position for just a few seconds may feel like a stretch, but it isn't long enough for the muscle to relax and lengthen. It is important to hold a stretch position for 30 to 60 seconds, about two or three deep breaths, and repeat the stretch two or three more times.

Stretching is beneficial to our bodies and especially so as we grow older. However, it is not a quick fix. It will take time to see the results of a regular stretching routine, but the benefits to your body and well being are worth it!

# Chapter 2

## Morning Stretches

Do you think it is too late to build muscle and Strength after 45? Well, if your answer is a "Yes," then you might want to rethink your response in a bit!

The actual truth is that age-related changes like slower metabolism rate, shrinking of your muscle mass, and the decline of hormonal and neurological responses are bound to begin at middle age. That's precisely how our bodies are built. However, when you begin to focus on improving your fitness performance, primarily through strength training, then, believe me, magic will happen!

Working consistently and diligently towards building and maintaining your body strength comes with many beneficial packages. It helps you keep your bones healthy, thereby reducing pain from arthritis which most seniors tend to deal with as they grow older. You can also easily improve your body's mobility and stability while working your legs to prevent occasional falls and hip fractures common with older people. Being regularly active also transforms to a lowered risk of several chronic conditions and illnesses. Now you can see that exercising can be a fun and rewarding way to stay active even as a senior. Fortunately, you don't have to spend hundreds of dollars on a lengthy course to get all these benefits. This book has compiled 101 highly-effective strength training exercises that can help you reach the highest point of your fitness performance.

This book is also designed to be your ultimate guide as you begin your quest to build muscle and Strength in almost the same way younger people do. At this point, I wish you a lovely time as you read and internalize the contents of this book!

101 Workouts to Improve Balance and Stability, Restore Strength, and Enjoy an Active Lifestyle

Before getting started with any of the exercises that we will soon be discussing, let's talk about some tips that will surely help you as seniors.

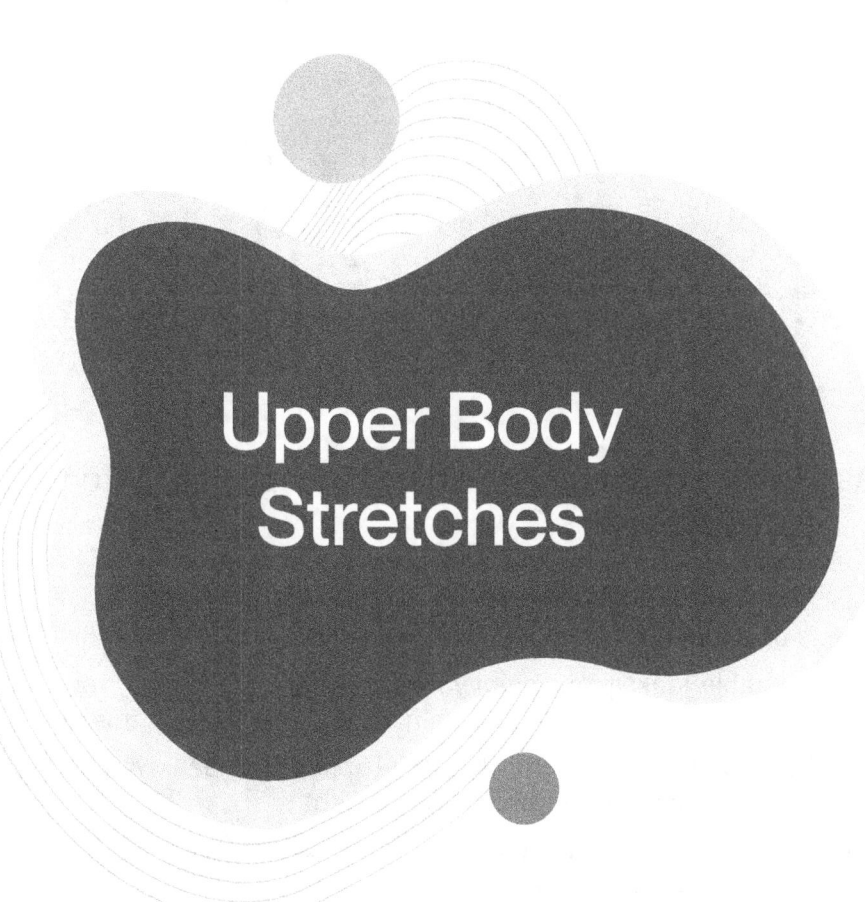

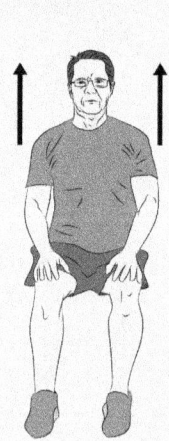 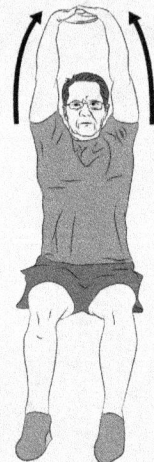

# Overhead Stretch

**Areas Stretched: Chest, Shoulders, Triceps, Lats, Front Of Neck.**

1. Standing with feet about hips width apart, raise both arms above your head.
2. Reach fingers, hands, and arms up as if you are trying to touch the ceiling. Take a deep breath in and then exhale.
3. If comfortable, look up and point your chin straight in front of you. Deep breath and exhale. If you have any neck pain or neck issues, skip this step.
4. With hands still raised, slightly bend the upper body backwards and hold for 2 or 3 seconds, then return to standing straight.
5. Lower arms back down to sides.
6. Repeat the stretch two or three times.

### Take Note:

- This can be done seated if you are unsteady on your feet or if you have any vertigo or balance issues.

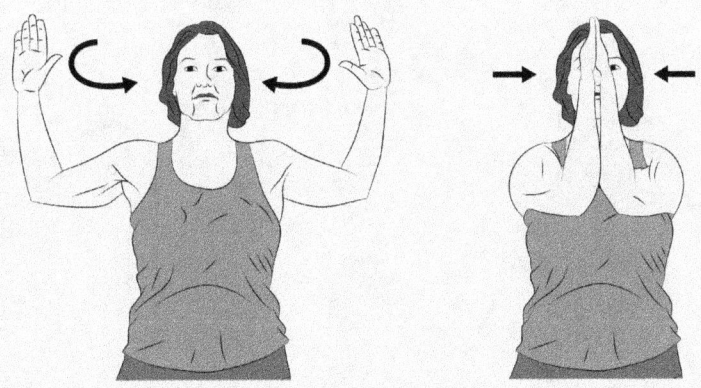

# Cactus Arms

**Areas Stretched: Front Of The Shoulder, Chest.**

1. From a standing or seated position, raise arms overhead and then lower to bend at the elbow to form 90 degree angles, palms facing forward. Your arms should form a cactus or football goal post shape.
2. With arms still raised and bent, push your chest forward as you push your arms slightly backward. Take a deep breath, then exhale and bring your chest and arms back to normal.
3. Repeat two or three times.

### Take Note:

- Protect your lower back if you are standing or sitting by not arching your lower back while doing this stretch. If you find you are arching, you can do this stretch lying on your back and taking care to keep your lower back pressed to the floor.

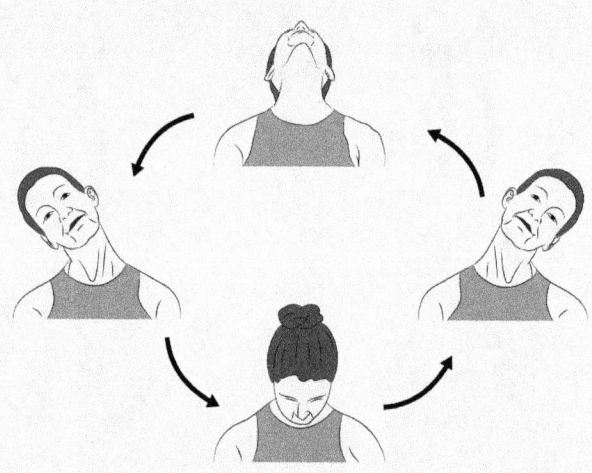

# Neck Roll Stretch

**Areas Stretched: Back And Sides Of Neck, Trapezius.**

1. From a standing or seated position, look straight ahead. Slowly tilt your head to the left as if your left ear was trying to touch the top of your left shoulder. Be sure your shoulders do not hunch up! Keep them relaxed and down. Take a deep breath in and then exhale.
2. Slowly roll your head down so that your chin is pointing towards your chest. Remember to keep the shoulders relaxed. Deep breath in and then exhale.
3. Roll your head to the right. Your right ear should be facing down as if to touch the top of your right shoulder. Deep breath in and then exhale. Slowly bring the head back to a neutral upright position. You can use your hands to gently help your head come back to upright.
4. Repeat two or three times. You can alternate sides by starting with the right side first.

### Take Note:

- Never tilt your head back while doing neck rolls. This puts a lot of unnecessary compression on your neck and spine.

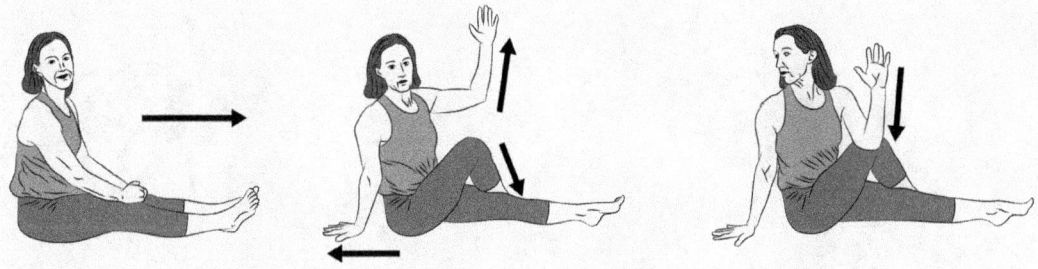

# Seated Spinal Twist

**Areas Stretched: Entire Back, Upper Glutes.**

1. Sitting on the floor cross legged, sit up tall and gently twist your upper body to the right. Place your left hand on your right knee and your right hand on the floor behind you.
2. If you can, look to the back over your right shoulder. If not, keep your head relaxed and look ahead or down. Take a deep breath in, then exhale.
3. Return your upper body and head back to the front. Take a deep breath in, then exhale.
4. Change the cross of your legs, now putting the other leg in front.
5. Sit up tall and gently twist your upper body to the left. Place your right hand on your left knee and your left hand on the floor behind you.
6. Look to the back over your left shoulder, if possible. Otherwise, relax your neck and look ahead or down. Take a deep breath in, and then exhale.
7. Return your upper body and head back to the front. Repeat the stretch two or three more times.

### Take Note:

- Keep both glutes firmly on the ground. If one side is lifting up, you are twisting too far. Only twist as far as you are comfortable.

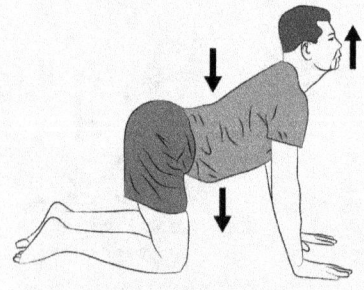 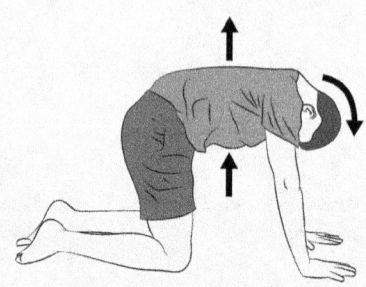

# Cat and Cow

**Areas Stretched: Upper Back, Mid Back, Back Of Neck, Shoulders.**

1. Get on your hands and knees on the floor. Your hands should be directly under your shoulders and your knees directly under your hips. Your back should be neutral and roughly parallel to the floor.
2. Take a deep breath and inhale while gently lifting your head and your tailbone. Your back will arch slightly and your belly will hang and be loose. This is called the cow stretch.
3. While exhaling, gently lower your chin towards your chest as you round your upper back towards the ceiling. Keep your tailbone and your abdominals tucked in but don't clench them. This portion is called the cat stretch.
4. Repeat the cow and cat stretches slowly, flowing from one to the other, several times.

### Take Note:

- Keep your shoulders away from your ears and relaxed while doing this stretch. There should not be any tension in your neck or shoulders.
- If your wrists cannot support you, a variation of this stretch can be done seated. Sit cross legged and place your hands on your knees while doing the cat and cow stretches.

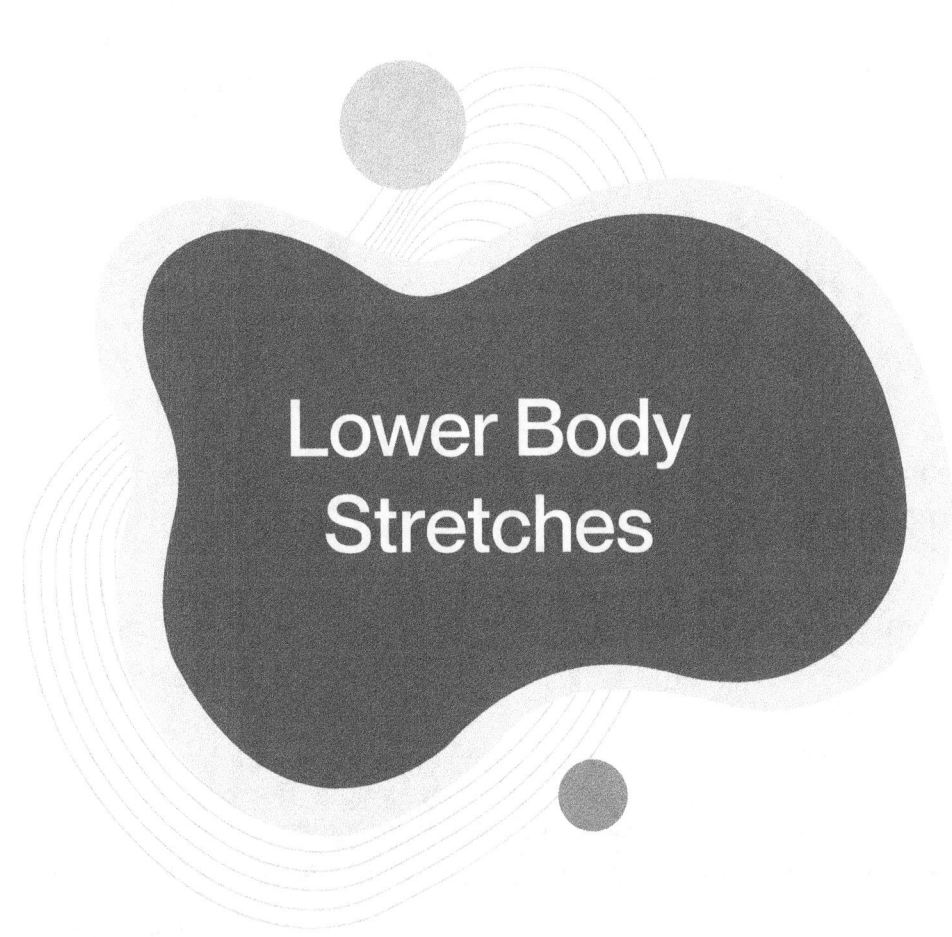

# Lower Body Stretches

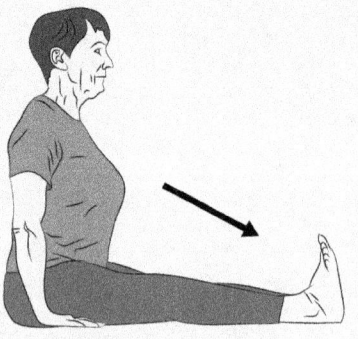
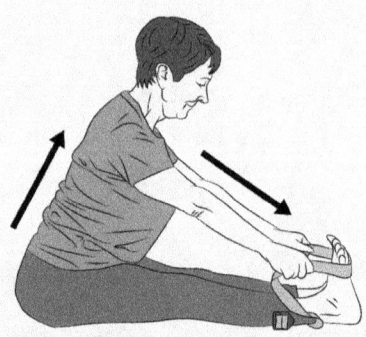

# Seated Forward Bend

**Areas Stretched: Entire Back Of Body Including Calves, Hamstrings, And Back.**

1. Sit on the floor with your legs together and straight out in front of you. Legs can be slightly apart.
2. Raise both arms overhead with palms facing each other. Take a deep breath in and then exhale.
3. While exhaling, bend your upper body forward from the hip joint. Keep your neck in a neutral position and your back straight. It is okay to have a slight bend at your knees; they don't have to be perfectly straight
4. Bring your arms down and let hands rest on the floor with palms facing up.
5. Repeat the stretch by raising arms overhead and starting again. Do this two or three more times.

### Take Note:

- Remember not to bounce when folding forward and don't force yourself to try to go lower. Hamstrings and calves are naturally tight in the morning. This should be a fairly passive stretch that just loosens up the back of the legs and back.

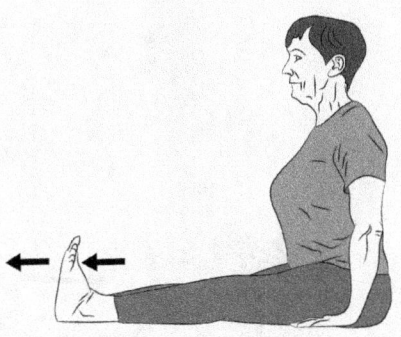
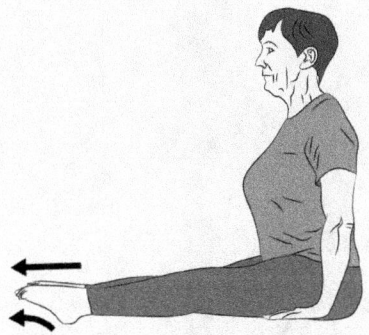

# Foot Point and Flex

**Areas Stretched: Toes, Feet, Ankles, Calves.**

1. In a seated position on the floor with your legs straight out in front of you, point the feet and toes. Stretch them as far away from you as you can. Take a deep breath in and then exhale.
2. In the same seated position, flex your feet and toes back so that toes point up to the ceiling and maybe even flex towards you. Take a deep breath in and then exhale.
3. Repeat the stretch two or three more times.

**Take Note:**

- This stretch can be done seated in a chair if the floor is too uncomfortable. You can also stretch one foot at a time if you find it too hard to do both feet at the same time.

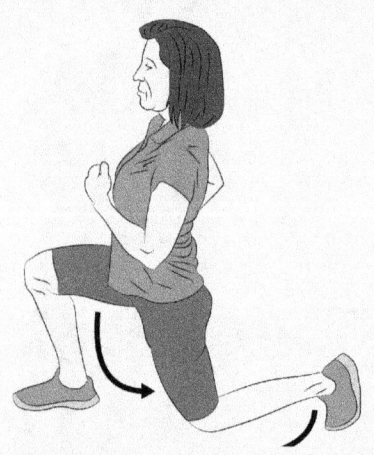 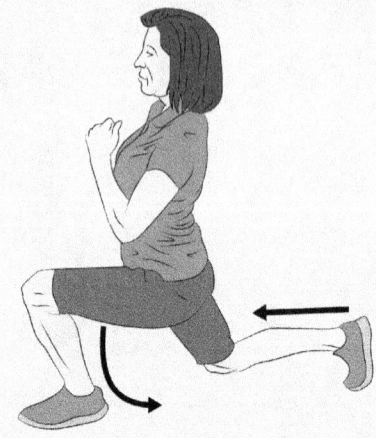

# Half Kneeling Hip Flexor Stretch

**Areas Stretched: Hip Flexor, Quads.**

1. Start on the floor by coming down on all fours with both hands and both knees on the ground. Get into a half kneeling position by lifting the left knee and bringing the left foot forward in front of you. Left foot should be directly under the left knee.
2. Raise up so that your body is upright and your right knee is on the ground directly below your right hip. Both knees should be at a 90 degree angle and hands on your hips. Take a deep breath in and exhale.
3. While exhaling, move hips forward. Your weight will transfer to your left foot and you will feel the front of your right hip stretch. Keep an upright posture. Take a deep breath in and then exhale. Move hips back to starting position.
4. Repeat the stretch two or three more times on the same leg. Switch legs to stretch your other hip flexor.

**Take Note:**

- Hip flexors are tight in most people and that contributes to back pain. Take this stretch slowly and allow your hip flexor to relax. As you do this stretch more regularly, you will be able to come forward farther.
- If you are stable and confident in this stretch, you can make it more challenging by lifting your arms above your head while stretching.

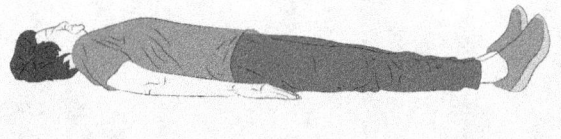
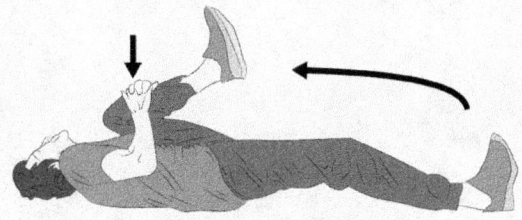

# Lying Knees to Chest

**Areas Stretched: Lower Back, Hips, Glutes, Hamstrings.**

1. Lie down on your back, resting your legs and arms on the floor.
2. Bring your left knee up towards your chest and place your hands either on top or behind your knee to support your leg. Don't tug or pull on your leg. Take a deep breath in and then exhale. Return your leg to the starting position.
3. Draw your right knee up towards your chest and either place your hands on top of the knee or behind it. Remember not to pull on your leg. Take a deep breath in and then exhale. Return your leg back down to the floor.
4. Repeat the sequence two or three more times.

**Take Note:**

- Once you are comfortable and confident in this stretch, you can make it more challenging by drawing up both knees at the same time. Either place hands on top of knees or one hand behind each knee for support.

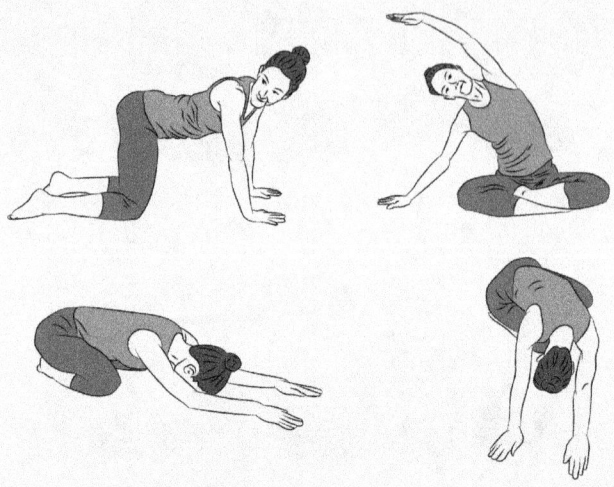

# All Fours Side Bend

**Areas Stretched: Sides Of Hips, Torso, And Neck.**

1. Get on all fours on the floor with hands directly below shoulders and knees directly below hips.
2. Pick up the left leg and bring it over the right leg and foot. Place the left foot on the floor as far to the right as you can comfortably get it.
3. Look over the right shoulder and back at your foot. Take a deep breath, lean into your left hip, and then exhale. You should feel the stretch along the entire left side of your body.
4. Bring the left leg back to the starting position. Breathe in and out.
5. Now, pick up the right leg and take it over the other leg and foot. Place the right foot on the floor as far to the left as you can.
6. Look over the left shoulder and back at your foot. Take a deep breath, lean into your right hip this time, and then exhale. Feel the stretch along the right side of your body. Bring legs back to the starting position.
7. Repeat the stretch on both legs two more times.

### Take Note:

- This is a deep stretch along the sides of the body and should feel good, especially in the morning. If you have neck issues, you don't have to look over your shoulder if it causes any pain. You can just concentrate on stretching the lower body.

# Evening and Bedtime Stretches

Stretching in the evening and just before bedtime is a wonderful way to wind down. Many people have a difficult time falling asleep at night. Sometimes the inability to relax before bedtime is related to our muscles feeling restless. If you have had a day of sitting in a chair at work, sitting in a car, or just sitting at home, your muscles need some movement and stretching to release the tension that has built up during the day. Along with releasing tension, stretching also increases circulation and blood flow to tense muscles (Sleep Advisor, 2020). Once the muscles have been stretched and relaxed, you will be less likely to toss and turn once you get into bed to go to sleep. This increase in the quality of your sleep is not only a benefit to you, but also to your partner who may awaken when you sleep restlessly.

When you relax the body, it's natural for your mind to also relax and get ready for sleep. By doing a regular night time stretching routine, your mind and body know it is the time that they can enter into a calming, loosening, and relaxing state. This focused state of deliberately relaxing helps you to separate the activity phase of your day from the restful phase of your night. Slow and deliberate breathing while performing these stretches also contributes to entering into a relaxed state. If you find that you are inadvertently holding your breath while stretching, you may be stretching too intensely or too fast. Your goal is to deepen and slow your breathing. Relaxing your body and your mind allows you to release the stress and tension of the day and leave it behind. This release may help you fall asleep faster and stay asleep longer.

If desired, you can take a warm bath or shower prior to performing these stretching exercises. This helps wash off your day both mentally and physically. It also adds a marker to your evening routine that signals to both body and mind that sleep is coming. Performing the evening stretches after a warm shower also warms up the muscles prior to stretching. Most of the evening stretches are done low to the ground and can even be done in bed, if you choose. If the stretches are done on the floor, do them on a padded mat or on your bedroom carpet. As always, look at your bed and surroundings to be sure they are safe to perform these stretching exercises on and use common sense.

Remember, you do not have to do every stretch in this chapter every evening. The goal is to unwind and loosen up, so choose one upper body stretch and one lower body stretch to do in the evening. Taking just five minutes to stretch before bedtime will help you relax before drifting off to sleep.

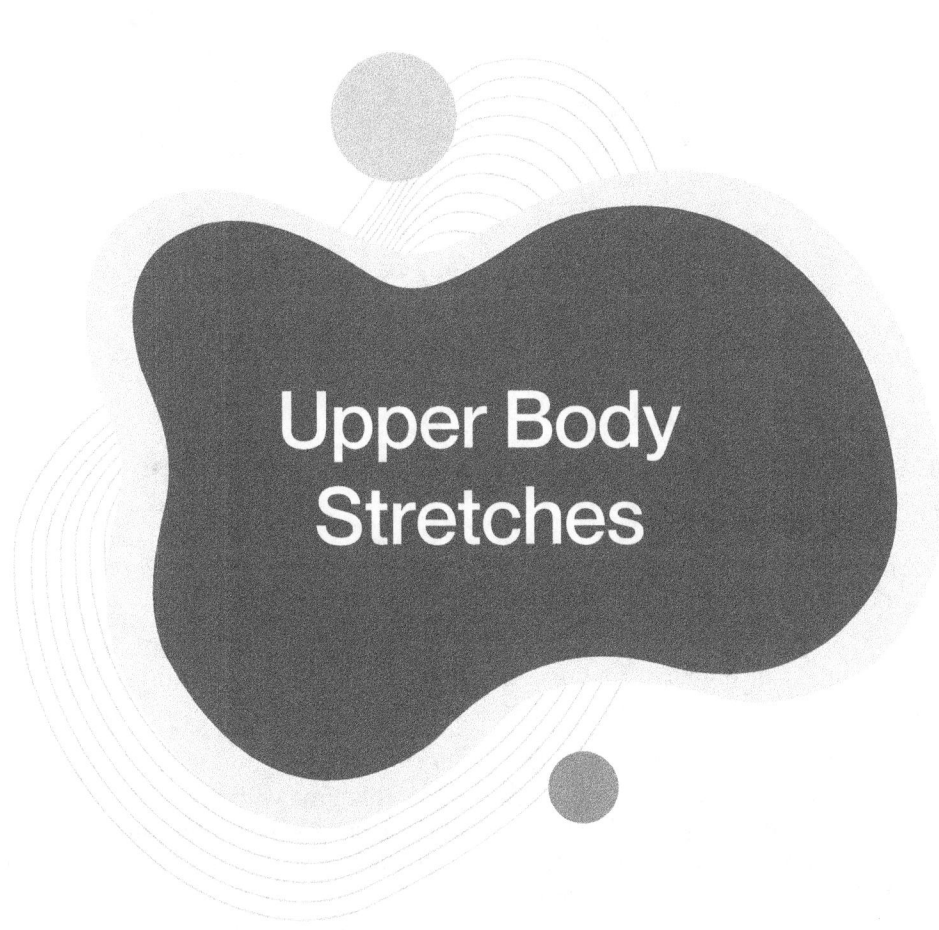

# Upper Body Stretches

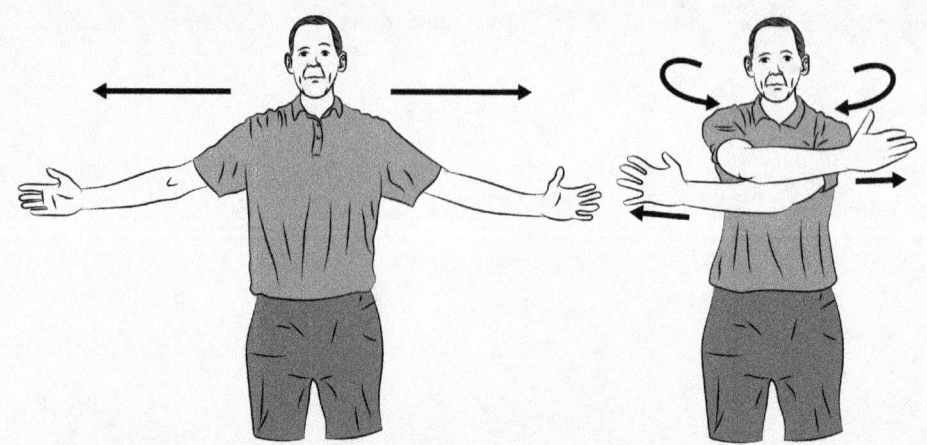

# Bear Hug

**Areas Stretched: Upper And Middle Back Including Trapezius And Shoulder Blades.**

1. From a standing or seated position, raise both arms out from the sides of your body, palms facing forward. Take a deep breath in and then exhale.
2. Take another deep breath in and gently cross your arms in front of you, right arm over left. Exhaling, give yourself a hug. Your hands should be touching the back of your shoulders. Hold this position and breathe in and out slowly two more times.
3. Release your arms and bring them back to your sides.
4. Breathing deep, gently cross your arms again, this time with your left arm over your right. Exhale and hug yourself. You may be able to bring your hands onto your shoulder blades, but if not just keep them on your shoulders. Hold this position and slowly breathe in and out two more times.
5. Release your arms. Repeat if you desire or move on to another stretch.

### Take Note:

- Depending on the length of your arms and the size of your chest, you may or may not be able to touch your shoulder blades. The goal here is to stretch the muscles of your upper back.
- Remember to not scrunch up your shoulders. Keep them down and away from your ears.

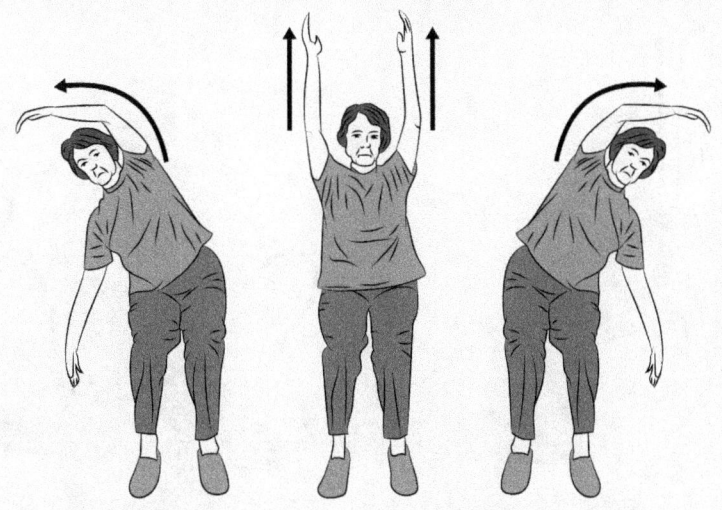

# Seated Overhead Side Stretch

### Areas Stretched: Entire Sides Of The Body, Neck, Upper Arms.

1. From a seated position, sitting cross legged, raise your left arm above your head and reach for the ceiling. Take a deep breath in.
2. As you exhale, bend your head and torso to the right while looking straight ahead. If it is okay for you, let your neck relax and allow your head to also bend to the right. You can place the other hand on the floor for balance. Take a slow, deep breath in and then exhale. Breathe in and out a couple of more times before returning to the starting position.
3. Change the cross of your legs. Raise your right arm up and reach for the ceiling. Take a deep breath in.
4. Exhaling, bend your head and torso to the left while keeping your gaze straight ahead. If possible, let your neck relax and let your head also bend to the left. Place your other hand on the floor for balance if you need to. Slowly breathe in and then exhale. Breathe in and out a few more times and then return to the starting position.

### Take Note:

- Don't allow your chest to fall forward or your shoulders to round during this stretch. Maintain good posture while doing this stretch by engaging your abdominal core muscles.
- Be sure to keep both glutes firmly on the floor. If one or the other is lifting up as you stretch to the side, you are stretching too far.

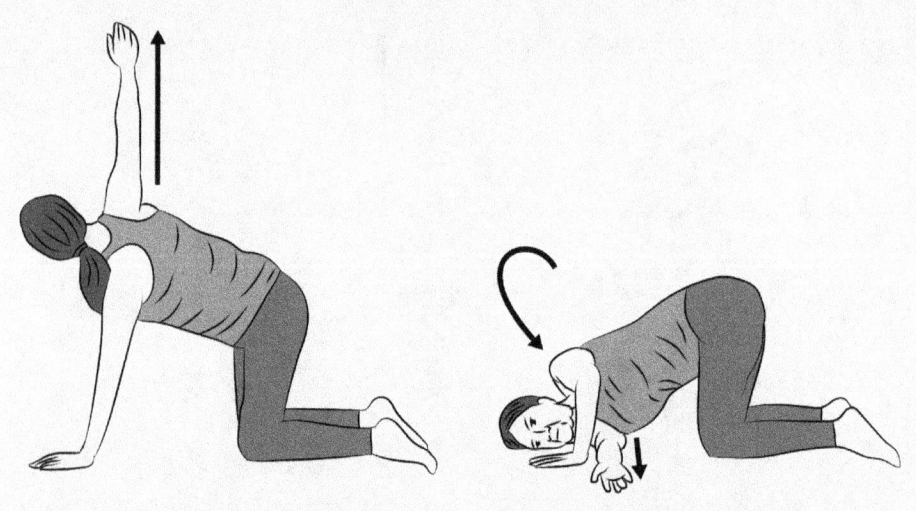

# Thread the Needle

### Areas Stretched: Shoulders, Upper Arms, Neck, Spine.

1. Get on the floor on all fours. Hands should be directly under your shoulders and knees directly under your hips.
2. Take your left hand and thread it under your right arm and just above the floor. Continue extending your left arm along the floor as you bring your left shoulder to the floor. Let your left hand rest on the floor, palm facing up. Your left ear should be resting on the floor as well.
3. Slide the other hand along the floor until it is above your head, palm down, so it is touching the floor just past your head. If this is too much, just leave your right hand where it is. Take a deep, slow breath in and then exhale. Your neck should be relaxed. Breathe slowly in and out two more times. Slowly lift your shoulder up and return to starting position.
4. To do the other side, take your right hand and thread it under your left arm. Extend your right arm along the floor and let it rest your hand on the floor, palm facing up. Bring your right shoulder down and rest it, along with your right ear, on the floor.
5. Slide the other hand on the floor until it is above your head, palm facing down. Again, if this is too much you can leave your left hand where it is. Take a deep breath in and then exhale. Be sure your neck is relaxed and breathe slowly in and out two more times. Slowly lift your shoulder up and return to starting position.

### Take Note:

- If this stretch is too much pressure on your wrists, you can start this on your knees and forearms on the ground. Continue the stretch by keeping your weight on your forearm as you slide the other hand and arm underneath the armpit.
- Depending on the strength of your lower back, you may need to avoid bringing your shoulder down all the way to the floor. If this is the case, you can place a pillow or cushion under your shoulder for it to rest on as you thread the needle.

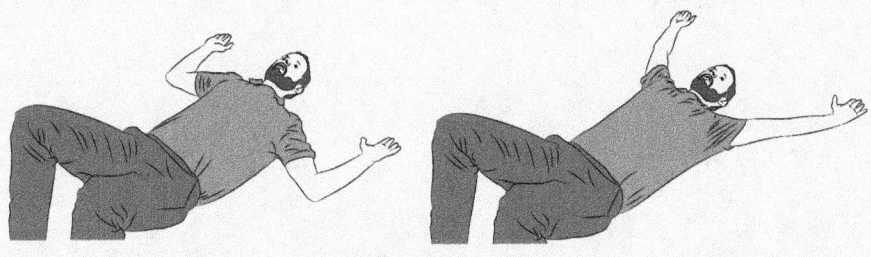

# Floor Angels

**Areas Stretched: Chest, Triceps, Lats.**

1. Lie on the floor facing up with legs straight and arms down by your side. Take a slow, deep breath in and then exhale.
2. Take a breath in while sliding your arms along the floor until they are above your head, palms up, just as if you were making "snow angels" in the snow! Stretch your arms and lengthen your body as much as you are able.
3. Exhale as you bring your arm back down to your sides.
4. Repeat the stretch two or three more times.

**Take Note:**

- Once you are comfortable doing this stretch, you can add your legs by sliding your legs apart as you slide your arms up.

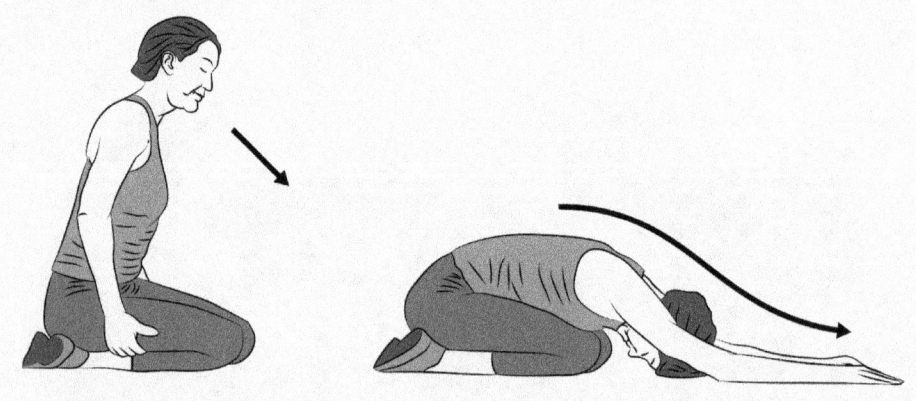

# Child's Pose

**Areas Stretched: Shoulders, Back Of Neck.**

1. Get on the floor on your hands and knees. Your hands should be directly under your shoulders and your knees should be directly under your hips. Take a deep breath in.
2. Lean back as you exhale and bring your glutes down and back to your feet. Lower your torso towards the floor and extend your arms along the floor up over your head. You should be facing the floor and your forehead may be able to come down to the ground. Stretch your arms as much as you can while breathing in deep. Slowly exhale. Take two or three more breaths in this position before returning to the starting position.

### Take Note:

- If your glutes cannot touch your heels, you can place a pillow or rolled up towel between your hamstrings and calves for support.
- Be sure to not scrunch up your shoulders when doing this stretch. Neck should be long and shoulders away from the ears.

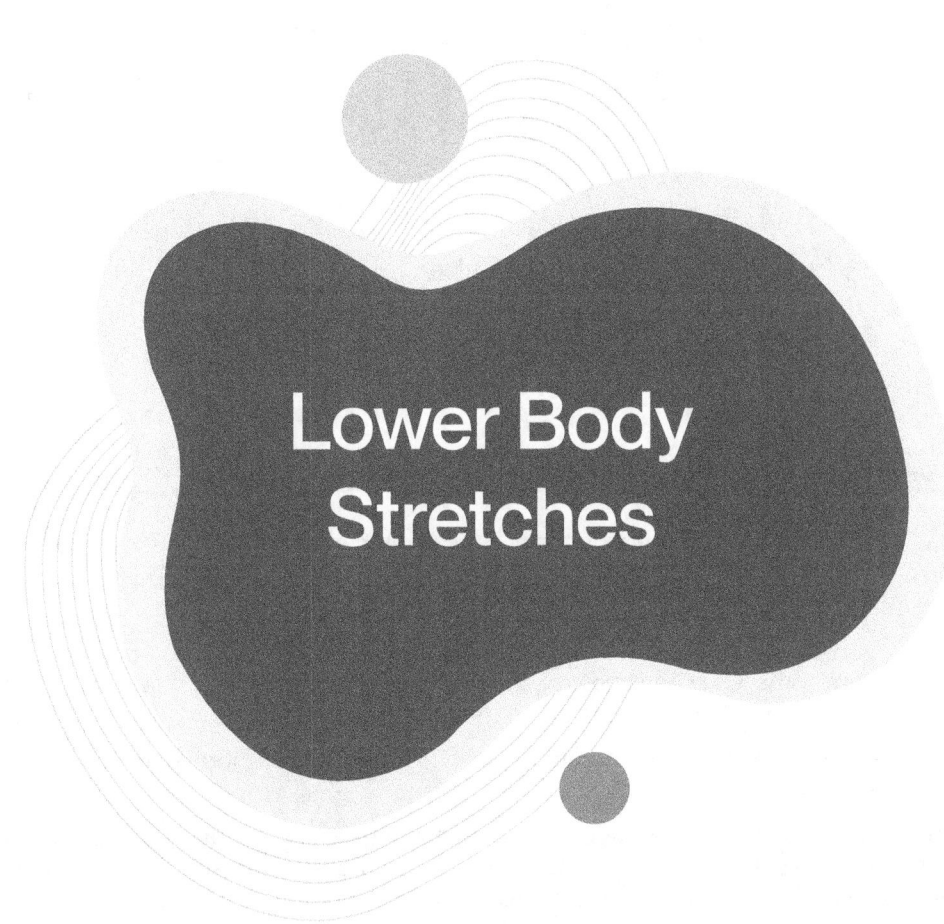

# Lower Body Stretches

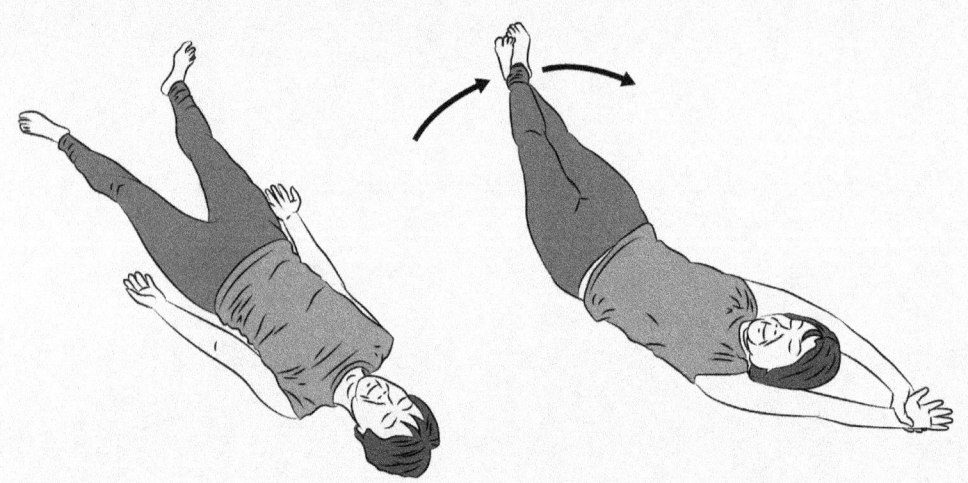

# Banana Stretch

### Areas Stretched: Sides Of Body Including Obliques, Lats, Hips.

1. Lie on the floor, face up towards the ceiling. Stretch your arms up overhead with your hands resting on the floor above you. Stretch your legs out straight. Take a deep, slow breath in.
2. As you exhale, slide your arms and legs along the floor to the left. If you can't do both at the same time, you can slide your arms first and then your legs. You should be in a banana shape and feel a stretch along the right side of your body.
3. Hold this banana shape and breath in and out slowly two or three more times. Return to the starting position.
4. To stretch your other side, slide your arms and legs along the floor to the right. Now you should feel the stretch on your left side. Hold the shape and breath in and out slowly two or three times. Return to the starting position.

### Take Note:

- You can deepen this stretch if you desire. As your arms and legs are sliding to the left, let your left hand grab your right wrist and gently pull. This increases the stretch in your lats and rib cage. If you are sliding to the right, your right hand will grab your left wrist.
- To deepen the stretch in your hips and IT band: as your legs slide to the left, cross your right ankle over your left ankle. If your legs are sliding to the right, cross your left ankle over your right one.

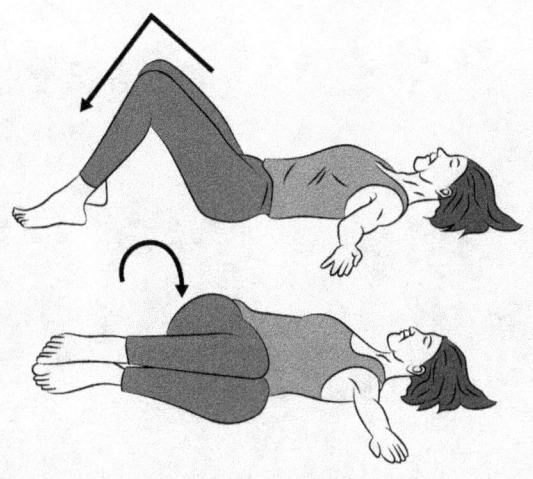

# Windshield Wipers Stretch

**Areas Stretched: Internal And External Hip Muscles, Tops Of Quads.**

1. Lie on the floor on your back, facing up. Bend your knees so they are pointing up to the ceiling and your feet are flat on the floor, hip width distance apart. Bring your arms out into a T-position.
2. Take a deep breath in. Slowly let both knees fall to the left as you exhale. Inhale as you bring your knees back up. Slowly let both knees now fall to the right and exhale.
3. Repeat the windshield wiper motion, left and right, slowly two or three more times.

### Take Note:

- Only let your legs fall to the side as far as it is comfortable for your hips. Keep your arms out in a T-position to help stabilize your torso as your legs go back and forth.
- A variation of this stretch can be done seated. Lean back and support your body with your hands behind you as your legs fall back and forth.

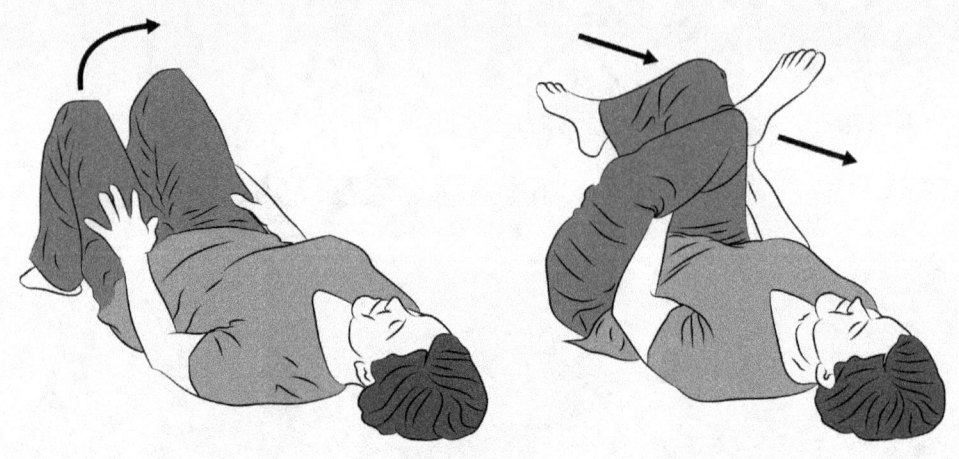

# Reclined Figure Four

**Areas Stretched: Glutes, Hamstrings, Hips, Lower Back.**

1. Lie on the floor, facing up. Bend your knees so they are pointing up to the ceiling and your feet are flat on the floor.
2. Bring your right leg up and cross your leg to form a figure four. Your right ankle should be resting on your left leg near your knee. Take a deep breath in and then exhale.
3. Let your hands grab behind your left thigh and bring your left leg towards your chest slowly and gently. Keep both feet flexed to protect your knees. Take a deep inhale and then exhale as you bring your feet back to the ground and uncross your legs.
4. To stretch the other side, bring your left leg up so that your left ankle rests on your right leg. If you can, grab behind your right leg this time and bring it towards you. Inhale slowly and exhale. Uncross your legs and bring both feet back to the ground.

**Take Note:**

- Depending on the mobility of your hips, just bringing your ankle up and placing it on top of your other leg may be enough of a stretch for you. Don't feel you have to draw the other leg towards you if you aren't able to.

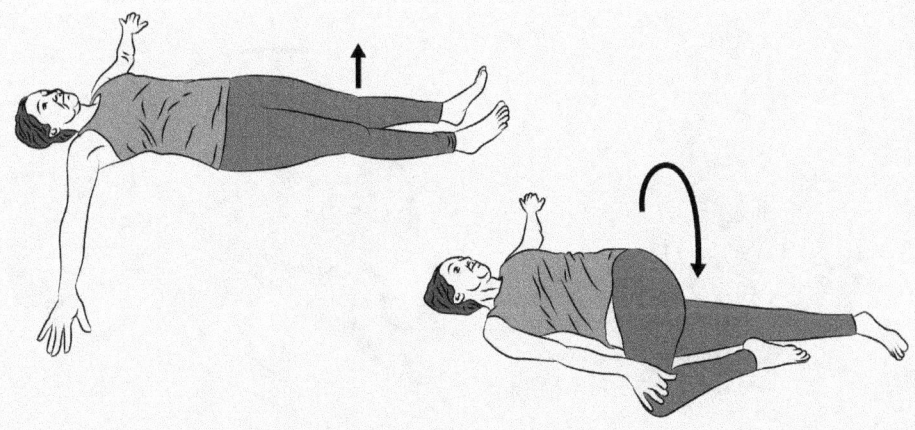

# Lying Spinal Twist

**Areas Stretched: Glutes, Obliques, Chest.**

1. Lie on your back on the floor, facing up. Bend your knees so that they are pointing up towards the ceiling and keep your feet next to each other. Bring your arms out into a T-position.
2. Taking a deep breath in. As you exhale, allow both knees to fall to the right until they reach the ground. Your hips should be stacked one on top of the other. If you can, turn your head and look to the left to get a neck stretch.
3. Inhale and then exhale as you bring your knees back up.
4. To stretch the other side, breath in and exhale as both knees now fall to the left until they touch the floor. Again, hips are stacked on top of each other. Look to the right if you can. Take a deep breath and exhale before returning to the starting position.

### Take Note:

- Don't force your knees to the floor. If you cannot twist that far, place a pillow or cushion to the side and let your knees rest on that.
- Both shoulders should remain flat on the floor and your chest should be facing the ceiling the whole time. If your shoulder is lifting up, you are twisting too far.

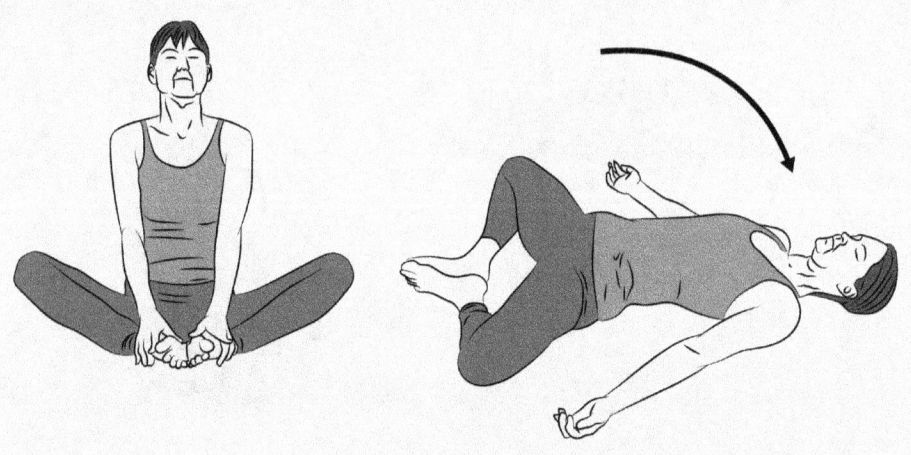

# Reclined Butterfly Stretch

**Areas stretched: hips, inner thighs, groin muscles.**

1. Lie on your back on the floor with your legs straight and your hands by your sides.
2. Take a deep breath in and slowly exhale as you bend the knees and bring the soles of your feet together. Your legs and feet should roughly form a diamond shape. Your knees may or may not touch the floor, depending on the mobility of your hips. Hold this position and breathe in and out slowly two or three times. Return to the starting position.

### Take Note:

- Depending on your flexibility, your feet may be close or far from your groin. Bring your feet to wherever is the most comfortable for you and your inner thigh muscles.
- For added stretch, you can slide your arms along the floor up above your head.

# Pre-Activity Stretches

Warming up before doing an activity gets your body and muscles ready for action. Just like you warm up a car in cold weather by starting it and letting it heat up to get the fluids moving, it's important to warm up your body to raise your body temperature and get the blood flowing to your muscles. You may be inclined to skip any kind of warm-up in order to get straight to your workout or activity, but you will be missing out on a crucial step and possibly jeopardizing yourself for injury. What are the benefits of warming up and stretching prior to a cardio workout, weight lifting, or sports activity? According to Cronkleton (2019), the benefits include:

- Lessened risk of injury because muscles are relaxed.
- Increased flexibility and ease of movement. Increased range of motion also reduces stress on joints and the tendons that support them.
- Decreased muscle stiffness because muscles are warmed up.
- Greater flow of oxygen and blood throughout your body and muscles because your body temperature has risen while warming up and stretching.

Most of us know to warm up before exercising at home or at the gym, but what about other activities? It's important for the muscles to be warmed up prior to every day activities such as biking, bowling, dancing, gardening, team sports, and even sex. Warming up by gradually increasing your heart rate and breathing allows your body to acclimate to the activity that it will soon be doing.

What is the best way to warm up and stretch prior to our activity? The American Heart Association (2014) recommends the following:

- Walk for five to ten minutes to get the muscles warmed up. An alternative would be to ride a stationary bike or swim for the same amount of time.
- Gradually proceed into your workout by doing whatever you plan on doing for exercise, but at a slower pace. If you are going to run, start off by jogging slowly.
- Incorporate movement into your stretches, but do not bounce. Stretch your entire body, both upper and lower areas.

Don't feel you have to do all the stretches listed in this chapter before your intended activity. Pick a few upper body and a few lower body stretches and do those. Next time, change it up and pick different ones to do.

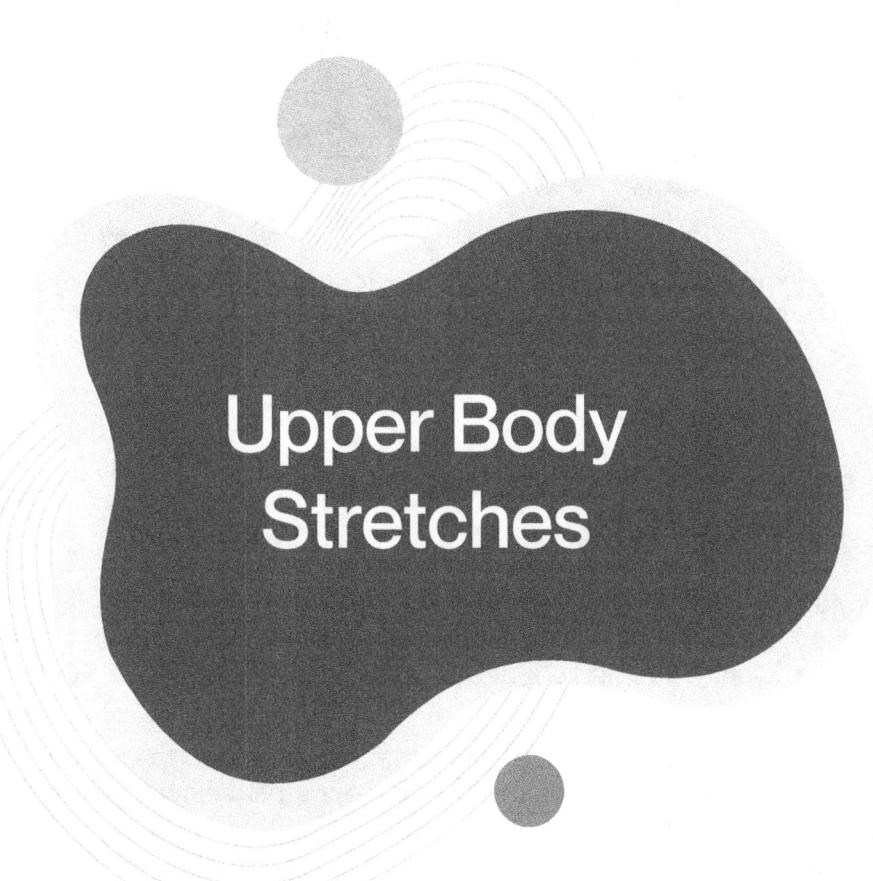

# Upper Body Stretches

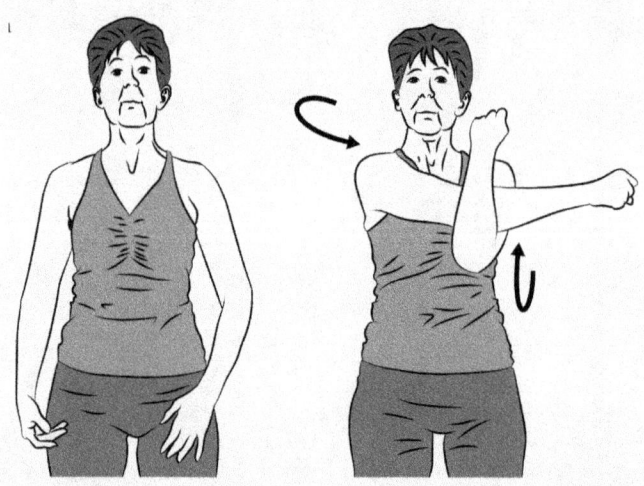

# Cross Body Shoulder Stretch

### Areas stretched: shoulders, upper back

1. Stand up tall with feet about hips width apart.
2. Bring your left arm up and across your chest to the right side. Support your arm by bending your right arm and letting your left forearm rest in the inside crook of your elbow. Take a deep breath in and then exhale. Return arms to your sides.
3. Next, bring your right arm up and across your chest to the left side. Let your right forearm rest in the inside crook of your other elbow. Breathe in and out. Return arms to your side.
4. Repeat stretches for both arms two or three more times.

### Take Note:

- Alternate support for the arm that is being stretched: stand facing a wall and allow your arm that is crossing your chest to rest between your chest and the wall.
- You can also do this stretch while sitting.

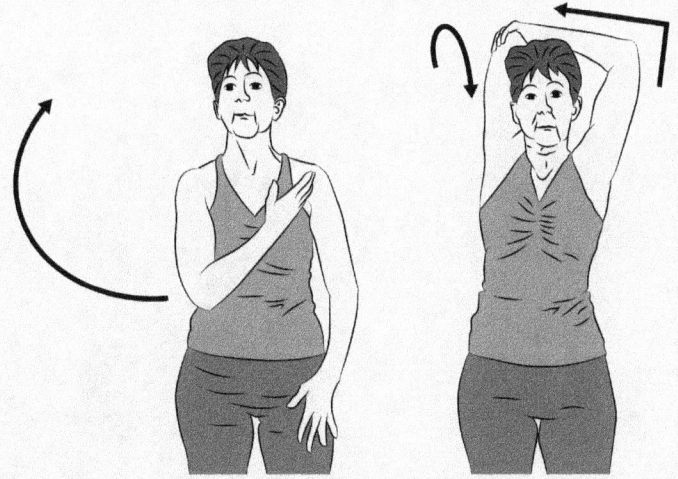

# Overhead Tricep Stretch

### Areas stretched: triceps.

1. Stand up tall with your feet about hips width apart. Shrug your shoulders up and then down.
2. Raise your left hand and arm above your head. Bend your left arm and place your left hand on the back of your neck or spine. Use your right hand to gently push your left elbow back as you slide your hand further down, if possible. Take a deep breath in and then exhale. Hold the position for two more breaths in and out. Return the left arm back down to your side.
3. Stretch the other arm by bringing your right hand and arm above your head. Bend the right arm and bring your hand to the back of your neck or spine. Use the other hand to push the right elbow back as your hand reaches further down. Take a deep breath in and then exhale. Hold the position for two more breaths in and out. Return the right arm back down to your side.
4. Repeat the stretch on each arm if desired.

### Take Note:

- Be sure to keep your hips tucked under you so you don't sway and arch out in your lower back. This stretch can also be done while seated

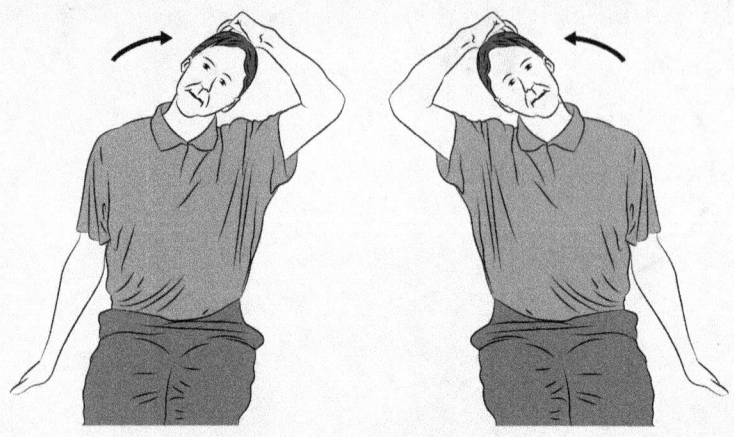

# Ear to Shoulder Neck Stretch

**Areas Stretched: Sides Of Neck, Tops Of Shoulders.**

1. From a standing or sitting position, look straight ahead and relax the shoulders. Shrug the shoulders up and then down.
2. While looking straight ahead, gently tilt the head so the left ear moves towards the top of the left shoulder. Take a deep breath in and then exhale.
3. Gently turn your head so you are now looking at your left armpit. Take a deep breath in and then exhale. Slowly return the head upright.
4. To stretch the other side, look straight ahead and gently tilt the head to the right. Your right ear will move towards the top of your right shoulder. Deep breath in and out.
5. Gently turn your head so your gaze now is towards your right armpit. Take a deep breath in and then exhale. Slowly return the head upright.

### Take Note:

- It's important to be very gentle and careful with your neck, especially if you have any neck problems or pain. Do this stretch slowly and deliberately, pausing when you need to. If looking down towards your armpit is too much for your neck, skip that part.

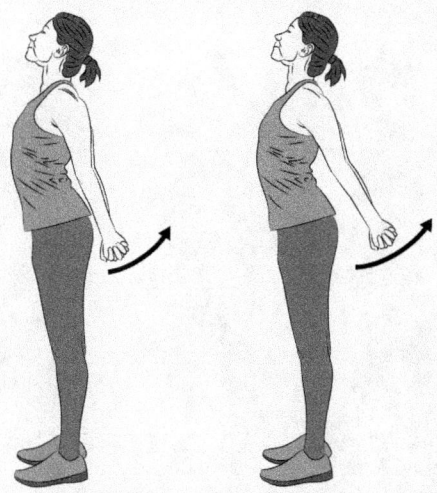

# Standing Chest Stretch

**Areas Stretched: Chest Muscles, Front Of Shoulders.**

1. Stand up tall with feet hips width apart and arms at your sides.
2. Bring your hands behind you and clasp them together and rest them on your lower back. As you take a breath in, push your chest out as you raise your clasped hands off your lower back and further out behind you. Slowly exhale. Hold the position for two more deep breaths in and out.
3. Return hands to starting position. Repeat the stretch two or three more times if desired.

### Take Note:

- Be sure you do not scrunch up your shoulders as you do this stretch. They should be down and away from your ears and your neck should be kept long and relaxed.

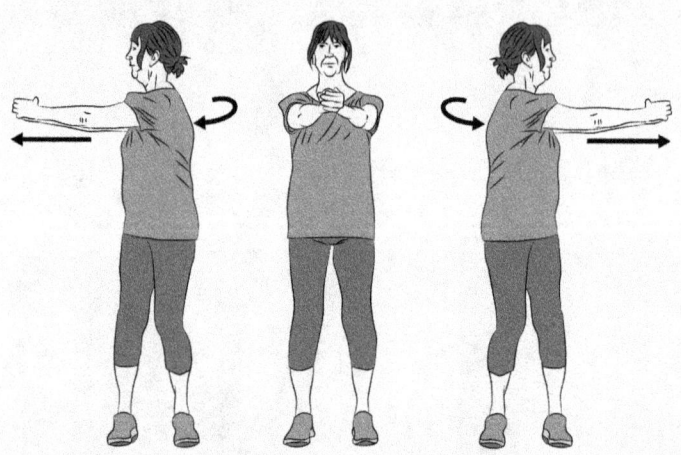

# Standing Torso Twist

### Areas Stretched: Abdominals, Obliques, Spine.

1. With feet about hips width apart, stand up tall with arms at your sides. Lift your arms up and out from your sides to form a T-shape. Take a deep breath in.
2. As you exhale, gently and slowly twist your upper body, including head and arms, to the left. You should be looking to the left and your lower body and hips are still straight ahead. Hold the position and breathe in and out. Return to the starting position.
3. To stretch the other side, breath in as you lift your arms up and out to a T-shape. Exhaling, gently twist your upper body, head, and arms to the right. Again, your hips should still be facing forward and your head should be looking right. Breathe in and out as you hold the position. Return to the starting position.
4. Repeat stretches on both sides two or three more times.

### Take Note:

- Don't be aggressive or jerky as you twist to the left or right. Protect your back and spine by moving slowly and gently.
- An alternate arm position is to bend your arms and bring your fingertips to the top of your shoulders as you twist.

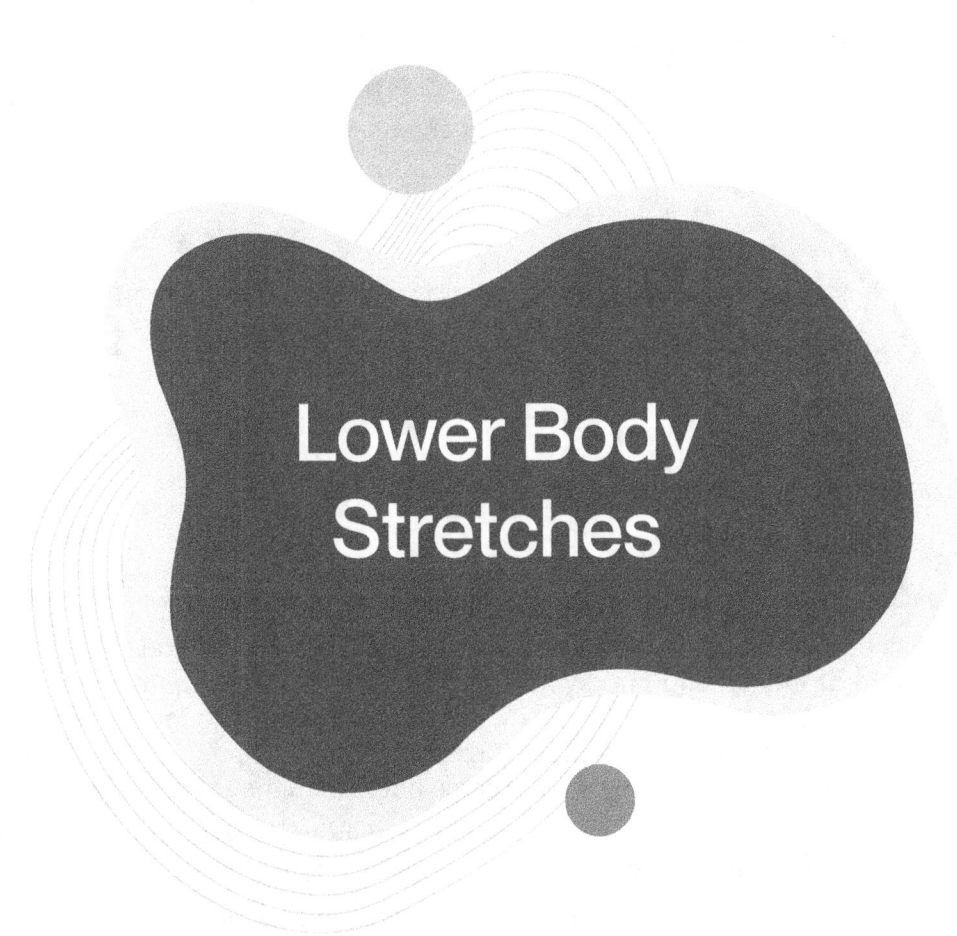

# Lower Body Stretches

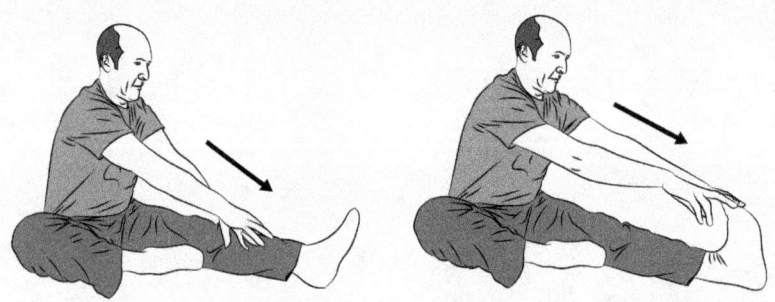

# Hurdler Hamstring Stretch

**Areas Stretched: Hamstrings, Glutes, Hips.**

1. Sit on the floor with both legs out straight in front of you. Bend your left leg and bring your foot to the inside of your calf, knee, or thigh.
2. Raise both arms up overhead and take a deep breath in. As you exhale, bend forward at the hip and bring your arms and torso down towards your knee. Depending on your flexibility, you may or may not be able to touch the floor in front of you. Take a deep breath in and exhale. Hold this position for two more breaths in and out. Raise torso and come back up to the starting position.
3. Switch legs by now bending your right leg and bringing your right foot to the inside of your calf, knee, or thigh.
4. Raise both arms up and breathe in. Bend forward towards your knee as you exhale and reach for the floor. Hold this position for two more breaths in and out. Return to the starting position. Repeat the stretch on each side two more times.

**Take Note:**

- Remember, don't bounce while doing this stretch and don't force your torso down. Only bend as far as is comfortable for your hamstrings.

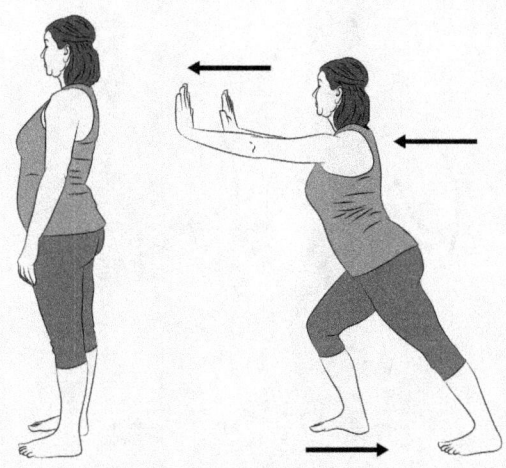

# Standing Calf Stretch

**Areas Stretched: Calves.**

1. Standing up tall with feet about 12 to 24 inches away from a wall or sturdy chair, place both hands on the wall or chair.
2. Lift left foot and step it back into a mini lunge while slightly bending the right leg. Press hands against the wall while you bring your left heel down to the floor, if possible. Take a deep breath in and slowly exhale. Bend your left leg to lift the heel off the floor and then try pushing the heel down to the floor again. Return to the starting position.
3. To stretch the other leg, lift the right foot and step back into a mini lunge while slightly bending the other leg. Press your hands against the wall as you bring your right heel down to the floor. Breath in and out. Bend your right leg and lift the heel off the floor and then push the heel down again. Return to the starting position.
4. Repeat the stretch on both sides two more times.

**Take Note:**

- Your heel might not touch the floor, and that is okay. The goal here is to stretch your calf muscles to a comfortable point.

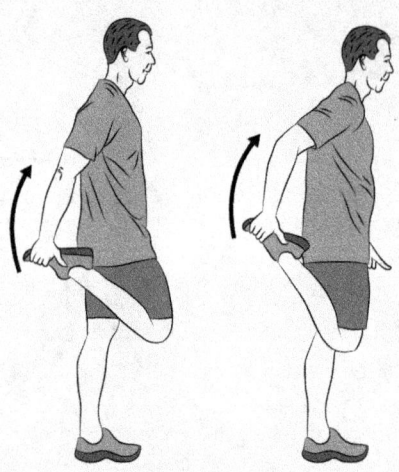

# Quad Stretch

**Areas Stretched: Quads, Front Of Hips.**

1. Stand up tall with both feet on the ground. If you need help balancing, you can place one hand on the wall or on the back of a sturdy chair.
2. Bend your left leg behind you and grab your left ankle with your left hand. Bring your heel as close to your glutes as you can without forcing or straining. Take a deep breath in and then exhale. Bring the leg back down to starting position.
3. To stretch the other leg, bend your right leg behind you. Grab your right ankle with your right hand and bring your heel as close as you can to your glutes. Breathe in and out. Bring the leg back down to starting position.
4. Repeat stretches on both legs two more times.

### Take Note:

- Be sure that you don't allow your lower back to arch. Keep the hips tucked under and pelvis facing forward.
- If you cannot do this stretch while standing, you can do it while lying on the floor. Laying on your left side, use your right hand to grab your right ankle. Lay on your other side to do the other leg.

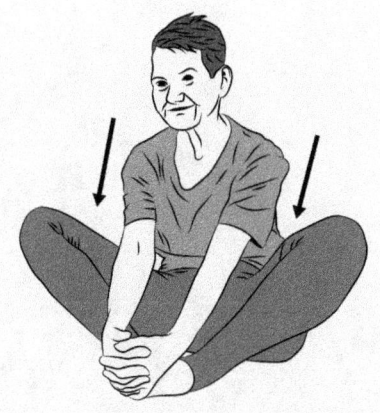

# Seated Butterfly

**Areas Stretched: Inner Thighs, Groin, Hips, Knees.**

1. Sit up tall on the floor with your legs straight out in front of you. Bend your knees out to either side and bring the soles of both feet together.
2. Slide both feet towards you as far as you can, keeping their soles touching. Depending on your flexibility, your knees may be either high off the ground or nearly touching the floor. Your legs make the shape of butterfly wings.
3. Take a deep breath in. While you exhale, bend forward and bring your hands to the ground in front of you as you lean forward slowly. Again, depending on the openness of your hips, you may or may not be able to touch the ground with your hands or lean very far forward. Breathe in and out two more times in this position.
4. Return to the starting position. Do this stretch two more times.

**Take Note:**

- If you are able, you can deepen the stretch by allowing your elbows to gently press down on your thighs as you are leaning forward.
- Don't round your back as you lean forward. Keep your spine straight, your neck long, and your gaze downwards.

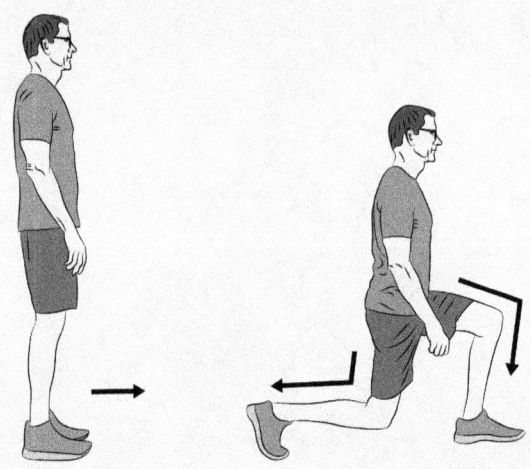

# Standing Lunge

**Areas Stretched: Hip Flexors, Quads, Calves.**

1. Stand up tall with your feet hips width apart. For stability and balance, you can stand next to a wall or sturdy chair for support.
2. Step back with your left foot behind you and bend your right knee. Your right knee should be directly over your right food and bent at a 90 degree angle. Keep your torso upright and do not lean forward. You should feel the stretch in the front of your left hip. Take a deep breath in and then exhale. Hold the position for two more breaths. Return feet to starting position.
3. To stretch the other leg, step back with your right foot while bending your other knee. Now you should feel the stretch in the front of your right hip. Breathe deep in and then out. Hold the position for two more breaths. Return feet to starting position.
4. Repeat the stretch two more times on each side.

### Take Note:

- Do not lean forward during this stretch. Keep your body upright and your pelvis pushed forward to ensure that your hip flexor is engaged and being stretched.
- Remember to keep your knee behind your toes so it stays at a 90 degree angle. Letting the knee come forward past your toes puts unnecessary stress on your knee.

# Post-Activity Stretches

Stretching and cooling down after participating in an activity is an important way to bring your body back to a normal state. Stopping suddenly after exercising or strenuous activity can cause your blood pressure and heart rate to plummet and make you feel as if you are going to pass out. When we exercise or participate in an activity that gets our heart rate up, our blood is pumping and our blood vessels are dilated to deliver blood and oxygen to our muscles. Coming to a sudden stop can cause a feeling of sickness and lightheadedness. Gradually ceasing the activity helps the body shift to a decrease in movement and exertion.

It is beneficial to stretch as the body is cooling down after exercise or prolonged activity. Your muscles are still warm and so are your joints and tendons. Stretching while still warm allows the muscles to stretch further and deeper, leading to increased flexibility and mobility. It is also good to stretch after activity to prevent the buildup of lactic acid in the muscles. Lactic acid builds up in muscles when there is not enough oxygen getting to the muscles. The result is stiffness and soreness in the muscles that can last for days. Stretching, as well as drinking plenty of water, helps prevent lactic acid build up (Cronkleton, 2018) by encouraging circulation and relieving muscle tension.

What is the best way to cool down and stretch, post-activity? According to the American Heart Association (2014), you should:

- Walk until your heart rate comes down (ideally below 120 beats per minute), about five minutes.
- Stretch the entire body, both upper and lower, and hold stretches for several breaths, about 30 seconds.
- Stretch deeply but not to the point of pain. Never bounce while stretching.

Cooling down and stretching after exercise and activity allows our bodies to recover and our heart rate and blood pressure to gradually return to what they were before we started our activity. Stretching while muscles are warm also prevents the blood from pooling in our lower body or other extremities after exercising. Plus, stretching after exercise or any activity feels good!

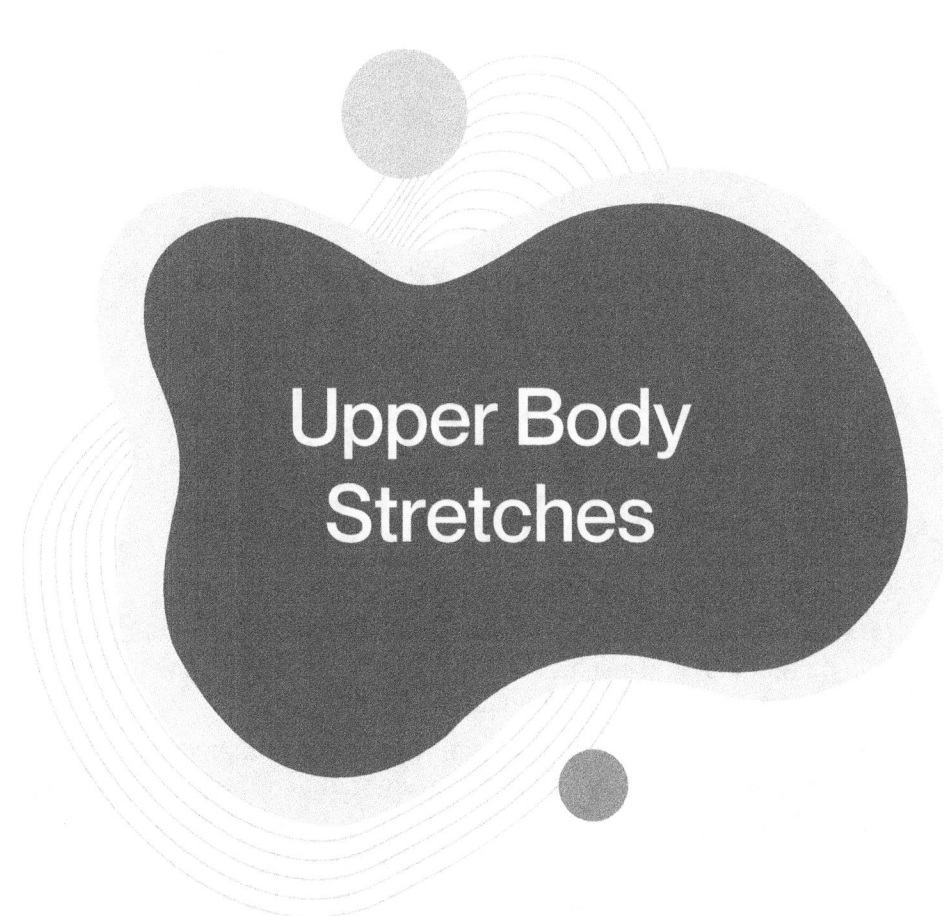

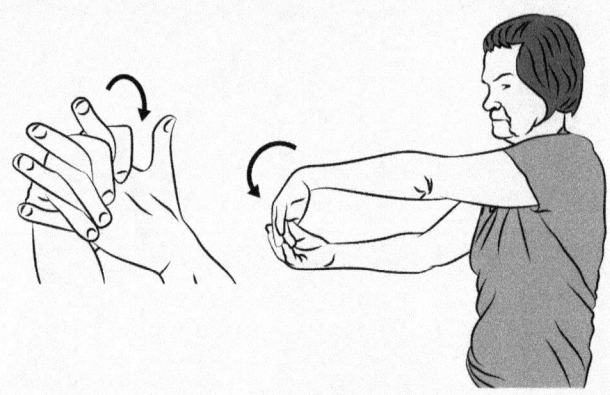

# Wrist Rotation Bicep Stretch

**Areas Stretched: Biceps, Thumb, Shoulder.**

1. Stand up tall with your feet about hips width apart. Raise your arms out and away from your sides into a T position.
2. With your palms facing forward, make each hand into a fist leaving the thumb free and pointed up. You will be making the "thumbs up" sign with both hands! Take a deep breath in and then exhale.
3. Now, rotate your wrists and arms so that your thumbs are pointing towards the floor. You will now be making the "thumbs down" sign with both hands. Breath in and out.
4. Repeat the stretch two or three more times going from thumbs up to thumbs down slowly and breathing naturally.

**Take Note:**

- Don't let your shoulders round and don't let your chest collapse inwards while doing this stretch. Keep your chest out and pushed forward for good posture.
- You can do this stretch while seated.

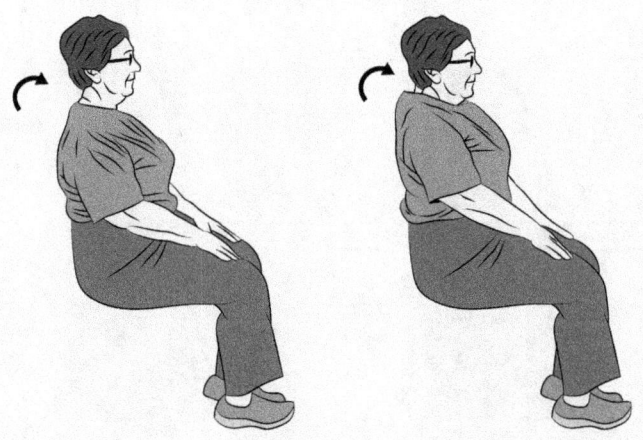

# Shoulder Rolls

**Areas Stretched: Shoulders Including Trapezius Muscles.**

1. Stand up tall with feet about hips width apart and arms hanging down by your sides.
2. Slowly raise your shoulders up towards your ears and then roll them back, squeezing your shoulder blades together. Breathing naturally, roll the shoulders up and back three to five more times. Return shoulders to the starting position.
3. Now roll the shoulders the other way by slowly raising them up towards your ears and roll them forward while rounding your upper back. Breathe naturally and continue to roll the shoulders up and forward three to five more times. Return shoulders to the starting position.

### Take Note:

- This stretch can be done any time your neck and shoulders are starting to feel tense. You can also do this stretch while sitting

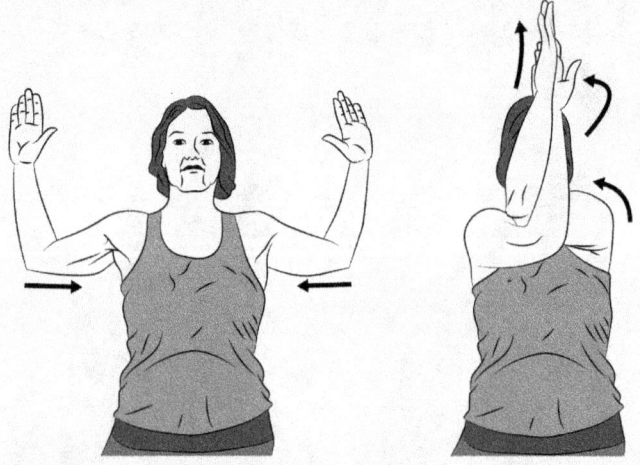

# Eagle Arms Pose

### Areas Stretched: Shoulders, Upper Back, Triceps.

1. From a standing or sitting position, bring both arms out in front of you and bend them so the elbows form a 90 degree angle.
2. Cross the forearms so that the right elbow is under the left elbow and the backs of your hands are touching each other. Raise your arms so that your elbows are about shoulder height. Take a deep breath in and then exhale. You should feel this stretch all across your upper back and shoulders. Slowly uncross forearms and return arms to your sides.
3. To stretch the other way, bring your arms out in front of you and bend them again. Cross forearms this time so that your left elbow is under your right one. Raise your elbows to about shoulder height and breathe deeply in and out. Slowly uncross forearms and return arms to your sides.
4. Repeat this stretch two or three more times.

### Take Note:

- Depending on the size of your arms and your chest, you may or may not be able to cross your forearms and get one elbow under the other. It is perfectly okay to just bring the forearms together and raise your elbows to shoulder height.
- Be sure to keep your shoulders down and away from your ears. Don't scrunch up!
- If you want to deepen the stretch, instead of just the backs of your hands touching each other, do another cross at the wrists and try to get your palms to touch each other.

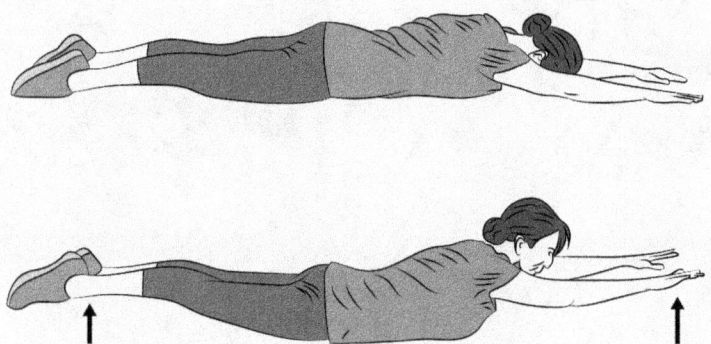

# Superman Stretch

**Areas stretched: upper back, shoulders, abdominals, spinal muscles, lower back, glutes.**

1. Lie on the floor, face and belly down, with arms out in front of you and legs straight.
2. Take a deep breath in and slowly raise your arms and legs off the floor a few inches and draw in your belly button. You should feel a contraction in your lower back and your body should look as if you are flying through the air like a superhero! Exhale and slowly lower your arms and legs to the ground.
3. Repeat the stretch two or three more times.

### Take Note:

- Keep your neck straight and look down at the ground, not straight ahead of you as that will put too much pressure on the neck.
- Lift your arms and legs only to where it is comfortable. If lifting both is too hard, just lift your arms.

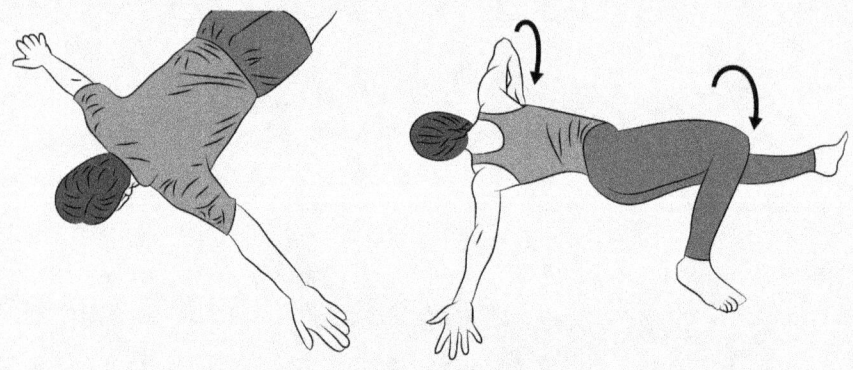

# Lying Pectoral Stretch

**Areas Stretched: Pectoral And Chest Muscles.**

1. Lie on the floor face and belly down. Legs should be straight and arms extended straight out to the sides away from your body.
2. Bend your left arm and bring your left hand on the floor just under your left shoulder. Take a deep breath in and while exhaling push into your left hand as you roll onto your right hip. Keep your right arm straight and extended out. You should feel the stretch in the right chest area. Hold this position for two more breaths in and out. Roll back to the starting position.
3. To stretch the other side, bend your right arm and bring your right hand under your right shoulder. Breathe in and exhale as you push into your right hand and roll onto your left hip. Your left arm should be straight and extended. Roll back down to the starting position.
4. Repeat this stretch on both sides two more times.

### Take note:

- Roll to the side only as far as it is comfortable for you. As you become more accustomed to the stretch, you will be able to roll farther.

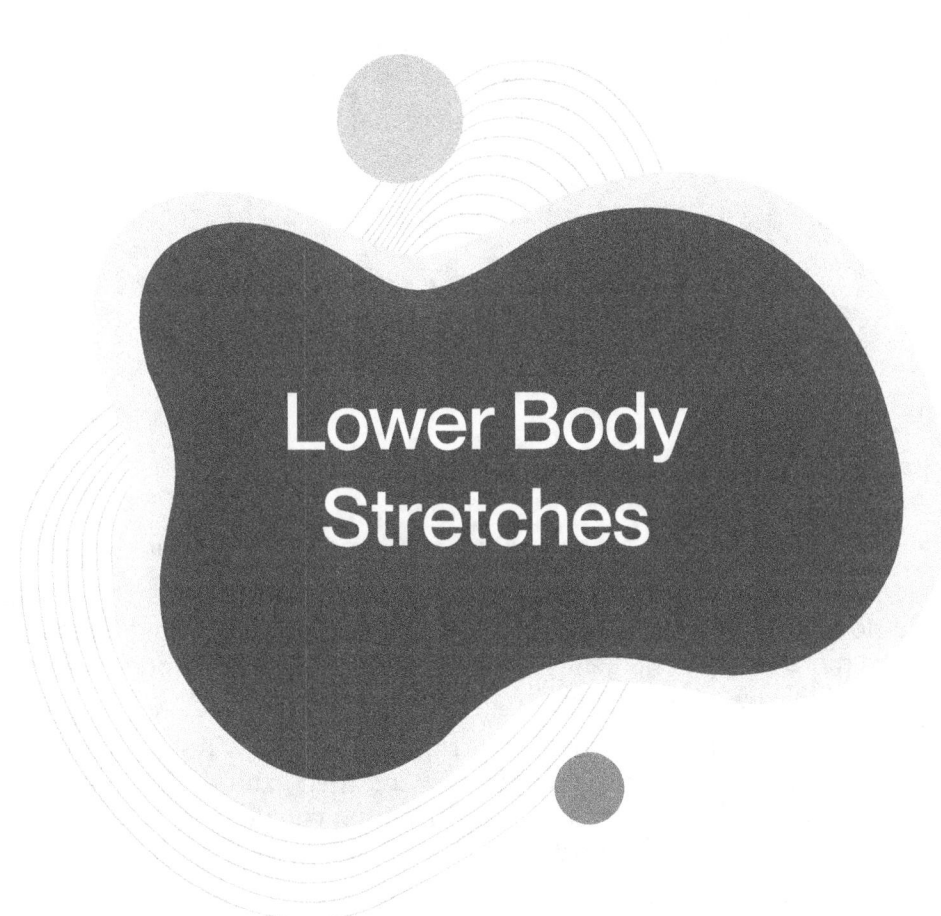

# Lower Body Stretches

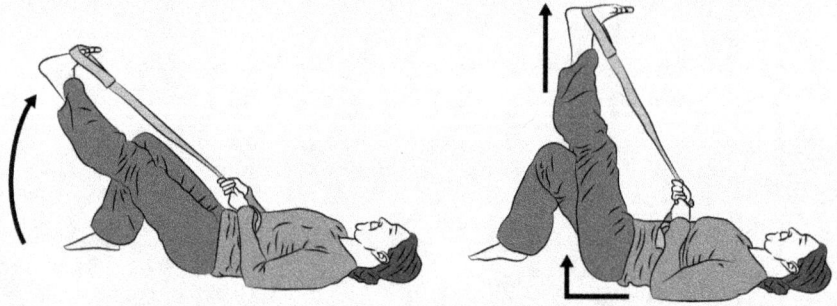

# Lying Hamstring Stretch

**Areas Stretched: Hamstrings, Glutes.**

1. Lie down on the floor with legs straight and arms down by your sides.
2. Raise your left leg and with both hands grab the back of your calf, knee, or thigh to support it. Take a deep breath in, and then exhale. Hold the position for two more breaths and gently bring your leg closer to your body, only if it is comfortable. Lower the leg back to the floor.
3. Stretch the other leg by bringing your right leg up and with both hands grab your leg where you can. Breath in deeply and then exhale. Hold the position for two more breaths and attempt to gently bring your leg closer to your body. Lower the leg back to the floor.
4. Repeat the stretch on each side two more times.

**Take Note:**

- Keep your head and upper back on the floor as you raise your leg to avoid straining your neck.
- If you are not able to grab your leg with both hands, an alternative is to do this stretch lying next to a wall, bed, or sofa where you can support the lifted leg.

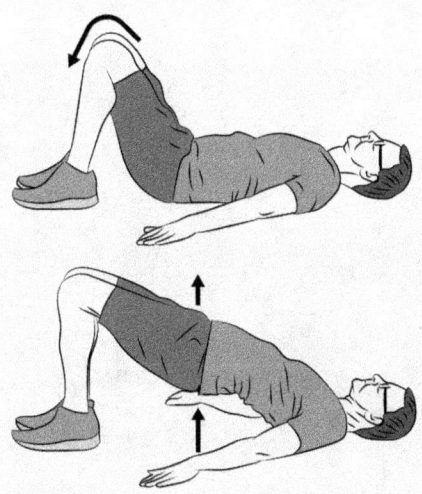

# Bridge Pose

**Areas Stretched: Glutes, Abdominals, Hamstrings.**

1. Lie down on the floor on your back with your arms by your sides. Bend your knees so they are pointing up to the ceiling and bring the back of your heels as close to your glutes as you can.
2. Take a deep breath in and exhale as you push your feet into the floor and lift your hips up and towards the ceiling. There should be a diagonal line from your shoulders to your knees. Hold the position while breathing normally for 30 seconds. If you can't hold your hips up that long, it is okay. Lower hips back down to the floor gently.
3. Repeat the stretch four or five more times.

### Take Note:

- Don't raise your hips too high. You want to avoid hyperextending your lower back. Your shoulders and hips should be in a line.
- Maintain good form when doing this stretch. It's better to hold the position for a shorter amount of time but correctly rather than holding it for 30 seconds incorrectly.

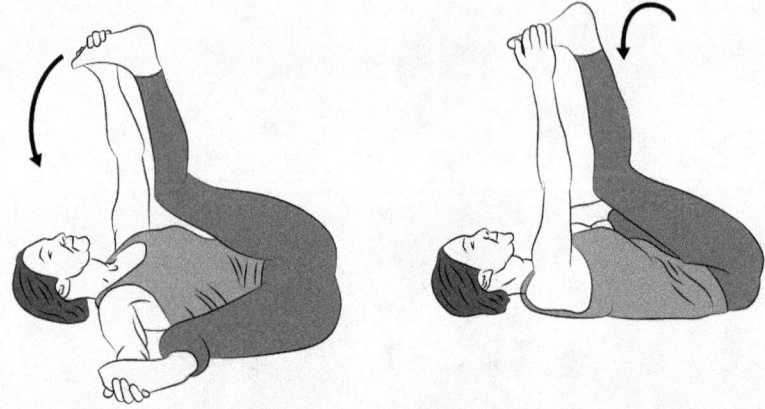

# Happy Baby Stretch

**Areas Stretches: Inner Thighs, Hamstrings, Groin, Lower Back, Hips.**

1. Lie on the floor on your back. Bend your knees and bring them towards you so your feet are facing up towards the ceiling.

2. Keep your head on the mat as you reach your hands up to grab your feet. You can grab the outer edge or inside arch of your feet, whichever is more comfortable for you. Let your knees fall away from each other and try to bring your knees to your armpits.

3. Gently rock from side to side, like a happy baby, while keeping your feet flexed. Breathe normally throughout the stretch. You can hold this stretch for several breaths, or whatever is comfortable for you.

### Take Note:

- Keep your head and shoulders on the floor for the entire stretch. Avoid straining your neck.
- If you cannot grab your feet without lifting your head or shoulders, try grabbing onto your ankles or shins instead.

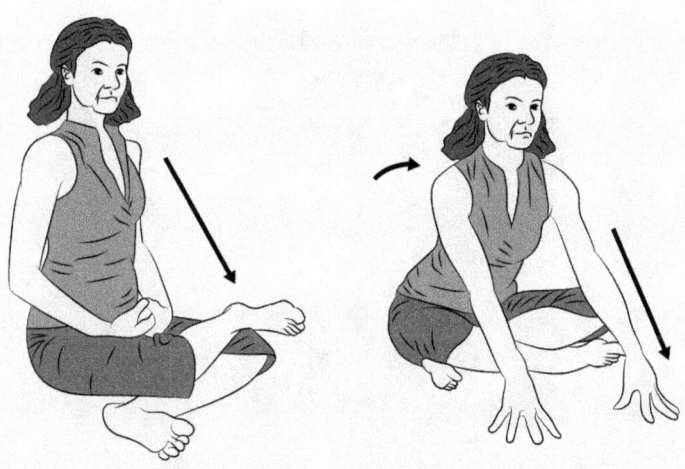

# Square Pose

**Areas Stretched: Hips, Inner Thighs, Spine.**

1. Sit on the floor. Bend your left leg on the floor in front of you so that your knee faces towards the left. Bend your right leg and put your right shin on top of your left. You should be sitting cross legged with your right leg directly on top of your left, shins stacked. Breathe in deep and then exhale. Hold this position for two or three more breaths.
2. To stretch the other hip, change the cross of your legs with your left leg on top this time. Left shin should be stacked directly on top of the right one. Hold this position for two or three more breaths.

### Take Note:

- If it is hard for you to sit upright in this position, place a blanket or towel under your tailbone for support.
- To deepen this stretch, fold your upper body forward using your hands on the floor for support. You can either keep your spine straight and long or round your back for a more passive pose.

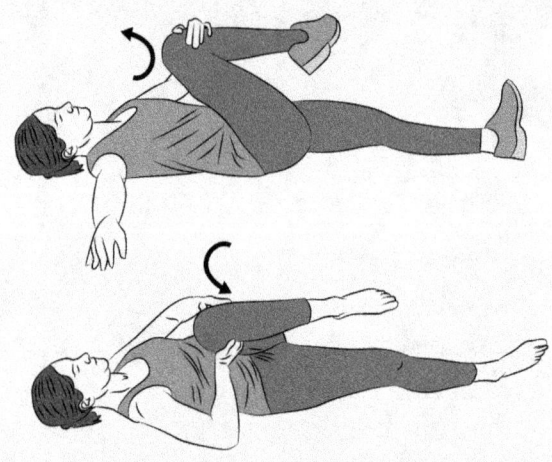

# Knee to Opposite Shoulder IT Band Stretch

**Areas Stretched: Iliotibial (It) Band.**

1. Lie on your back on the floor with your legs straight and arms by your sides.
2. Bend and raise your left knee towards you, grabbing behind your knee with both hands. Gently bring your knee towards the right shoulder. You should feel the stretch on the outside of your left hip and thigh where the IT band runs. Take a deep breath in and out. Hold the position for two or three more breaths. Gently lower the leg back to the starting position.
3. To stretch the other leg, raise and bend your right leg. Grab behind your knee and gently bring your right knee towards your left shoulder. Breathe deeply in and then exhale. Hold the position for two or three more breaths. Gently lower the leg and return to the starting position.
4. Repeat the stretch on both legs two more times.

**Take Note:**

- A tight IT band can cause pain at the knee and hip joints, so go slowly and carefully when doing this stretch. Don't jerk on your knee at any time.
- Keep your head and shoulders on the floor to avoid any neck strain.

# Chapter 6

## Target Area Stretches

In the previous chapters, we have concentrated on the large muscles of the upper and lower body. These are the muscles that contribute to our daily movement and mobility. There are many other muscles that can be stretched to relieve pain or to increase flexibility in a targeted area of the body. In this chapter, we will learn some stretches that work on some of the smaller, but no less important, areas that can benefit from a stretching routine.

The extremities, namely the hands and feet, are used daily and can become tight or stiff. Stretching the fingers, hands, and wrists helps with fine motor skills and mobility to do simple tasks like holding small items, writing, buttoning clothing, eating, using scissors, and even typing. The small muscles in our hands were designed to accomplish these fine motor skills. As we grow older, we sometimes find that our ability to do some of these skills diminishes because of joint stiffness and a loss of muscle flexibility. By doing a few easy stretches every day, we keep our joints and muscles moving and limber, allowing us to continue doing the activities that call for fine motor control.

Stretching the toes, feet, and ankles keeps us on our feet, literally. If you have ever experienced foot or ankle pain, you know how debilitating that can be to physical movement and even mental health. Our feet are subjected to daily pressure which is sometimes made worse by inflammation, conditions like plantar fasciitis, and even ill-fitting shoes. The benefits of stretching the big muscles in our arms and legs apply also to the small muscles in our feet. Increased blood flow and circulation brings oxygen to the muscles in our feet and allows us to stretch the muscles and elongate them, reducing pain and stiffness. The increased flexibility in our feet also aids us in our balance. This helps prevent falls due to imbalance.

These targeted areas are also areas that are prone to arthritis and other joint conditions, so if you have challenges with that check with your doctor, chiropractor, or health provider before doing these stretches. As always, use common sense and discontinue any stretch that causes pain at any time.

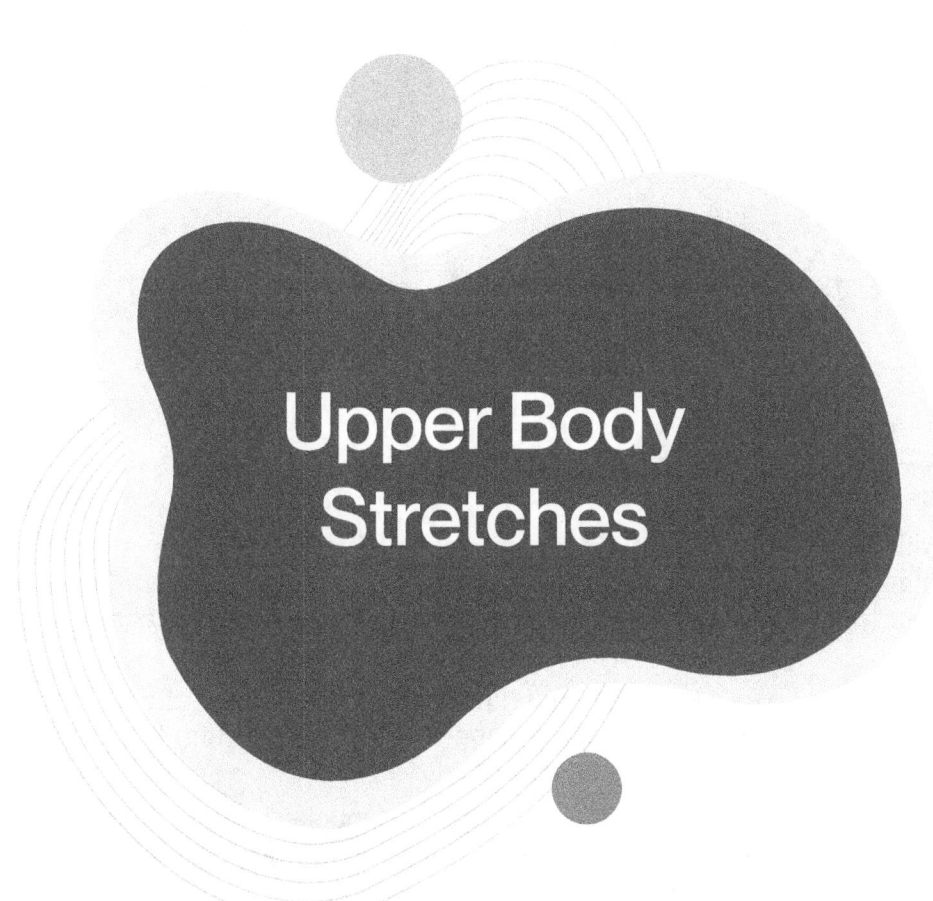

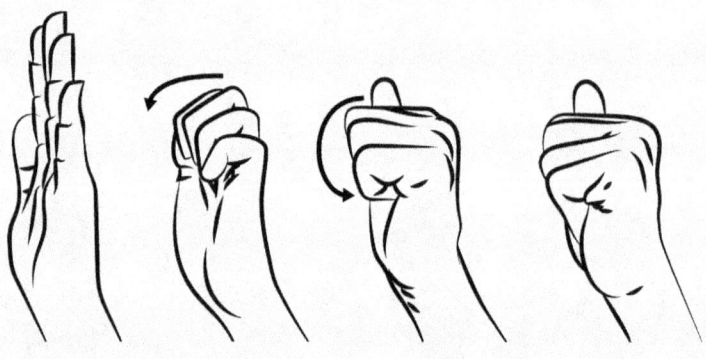

# Hand and Finger Tendon Glide

**Areas Stretched: Tendons In The Hands And Fingers**

1. With both hands in front of you and palms facing each other, straighten the fingers and thumbs. Slowly bend just the fingers until the fingertips touch the upper part of your palms. Hold the position for 30 seconds. Straighten fingers slowly.
2. Next, bend fingers until the fingertips touch the middle of the palms. Make a fist by bringing thumbs over the fingers. Hold the position for 30 seconds. Slowly straighten fingers and thumbs.
3. Finally, keep fingers straight and bend at the knuckle to bring fingertips down towards the bottom or meaty part of the palms. Hold the position for 30 seconds. Bring fingers back to starting position.
4. Repeat the three stretches a few more times. Breathe normally throughout the stretching.

**Take Note:**

- Depending on your finger and hand mobility, these exercises may be difficult for one or both hands. You can also do these stretches one hand at a time.
- Don't hold your breath or clench your jaw while doing these stretches. It can sometimes happen when we are focused and intent, so just be aware!

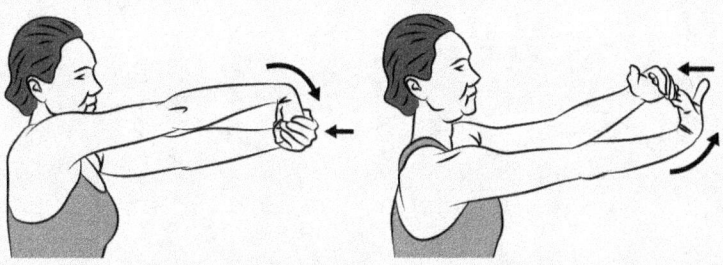

# Wrist Flexor and Extensor Stretch

**Areas Stretched: Wrists, Forearms.**

1. From a seated position, rest your left forearm on a table or countertop so that your elbow forms a 90 degree angle. Position yourself so that your left arm is next to your body with your left hand facing down and wrist hanging over the edge of the table. Slowly lower your hand so that your palm is now facing you and your fingertips are pointing towards the floor.
2. Slowly raise your hand so that your palm is now facing away from you and your fingertips are pointing towards the ceiling. Do this stretch both ways two more times, breathing normally while stretching.
3. Change positions so that now your right forearm is resting on the table with your right hand facing down and wrist over the edge. Lower your right hand slowly so your palm is facing you and your fingertips are pointing towards the floor.
4. Raise your hand slowly until your right palm is facing away from you and fingertips are pointing at the ceiling. Stretch both ways two more times while breathing normally.

**Take Note:**

- If needed, you can place a folded or rolled hand towel under your forearm for extra padding and support.
- A variation of this stretch is to form your hand into a fist with your thumb over your fingers. Lower and raise your fist slowly.

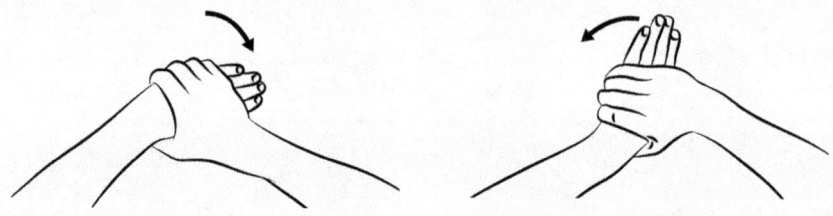

# Wrist Ulnar and Radial Stretch

**Areas Stretched: Wrists, Forearms.**

1. From a seated position, rest your left forearm on a table so that your elbow forms a 90 degree angle. Bring your left arm next to your body with your thumb and fingertips straight ahead with your palm facing inward. Slowly lower your wrist and hand toward the floor and then bring it up straight ahead and slightly towards the ceiling if possible, going through the full range of motion. Breathe normally as you repeat this stretch two more times.
2. To stretch the other side, change positions so that your right forearm is resting on the table. With your right arm next to your body and fingertips straight ahead, face your palm inward. Slowly move your hand and wrist up toward the ceiling and down toward the floor, through the full range of motion. Repeat the stretch two more times.

**Take Note:**

- This stretch uses different muscles in the wrist and forearm and you may not have the same range of flexibility as you do with other wrist stretches.

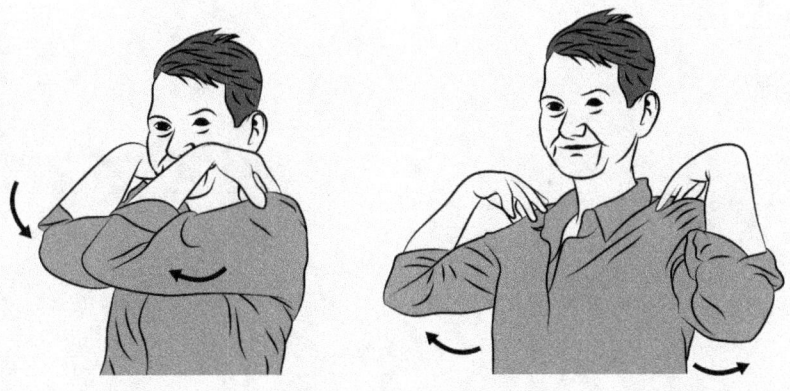

# Butterfly Wings Upper Back Stretch

**Areas Stretched:** Upper Back Including Rhomboids, Upper Chest Including Pecs.

1. From a standing or seated position, lift both arms and bend at the elbows. Allow the fingertips to touch the shoulders, left hand touches left shoulder and right hand touches right shoulder. These form the "butterfly wings."
2. Take a deep breath in. As you exhale, bring your elbows together out in front of you and try to touch them together. Be sure to keep your fingertips on your shoulders.
3. Gently bring elbows back out to sides and slightly behind you, if possible. Repeat the stretch both ways two or three more times, exhaling as you bring your elbows together.

### Take Note:

- Depending on the size of your chest and your flexibility, you may or may not be able to touch your elbows together. It's okay if they don't touch. Your upper back will still experience a stretch.

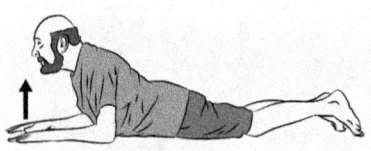 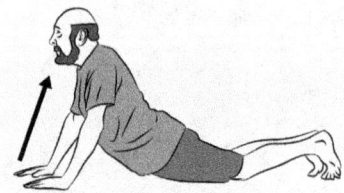

# Cobra Abs

**Areas Stretched: Abdominals.**

1. Lie on the floor, face down, with your feet pointing away from you. Place your hands directly under your shoulders.
2. Take a deep breath in. As you exhale, press down through your hands to raise your upper torso off the floor. Keep shoulders down and away from your ears while keeping your neck long. Hips and legs should remain on the floor. Breathe in and out once more and slowly lower your torso back down to the floor.
3. Repeat this stretch two or three more times, going slowly.

**Take Note:**

- Do not do this stretch if you have any back issues or severe back pain.
- Only lift up your torso as far as it is comfortable for you.

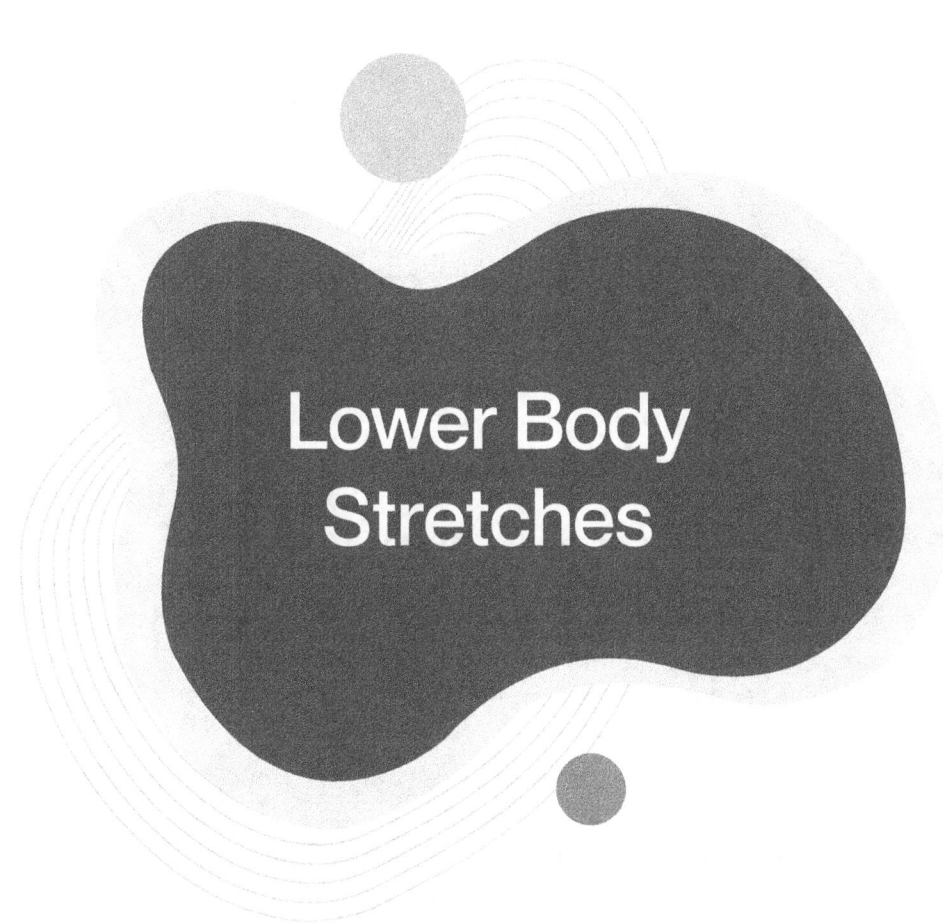

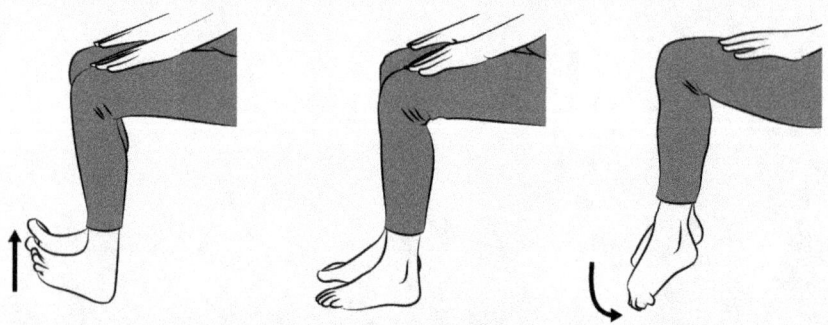

# Toe Raises, Points, and Curls

### Areas Stretched: Toes, Feet, Ankles.

1. From a seated position in a chair, place both feet flat on the floor. Keeping toes and balls of the feet on the floor, raise both heels so they are off the floor as high as you can get them. Hold the position for 15 to 30 seconds.
2. Next, point your toes, ballerina style, so that only the tips of your big toes (and possibly your second toes) are on the ground. Hold the position for 15 to 30 seconds.
3. Finally, curl your toes towards the soles of your feet. Now the tops of your toes should be on the ground and you feel the stretch in the front of your ankles. Hold the position for 15 to 30 seconds. Return feet to the starting position.
4. Repeat the stretches two or three more times.

### Take Note:

- If you have had any foot surgery, check with your doctor before doing these stretches.
- Breathe normally while doing these stretches and keep your shoulders down and relaxed. If you feel any pain while doing the stretches, immediately stop.

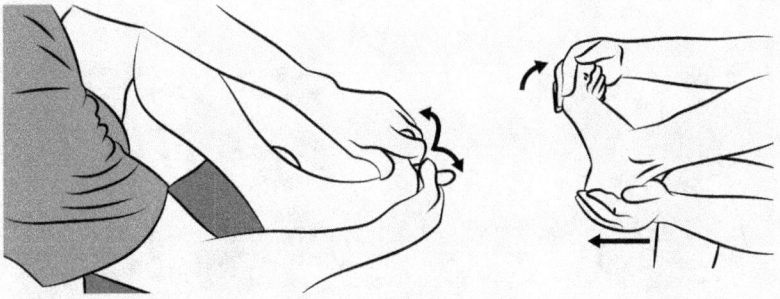

# Toe Extension or Foot Flex

### Areas Stretched: Heels, Ankles.

1. From a seated position, bring your left ankle up and place it on top of your right knee. Grab your left toes with your left hand and gently pull them up towards your ankle. You should feel the stretch in your heel and back of the ankle. Hold for two breaths in and out and return foot to the starting position.
2. To stretch the other foot, bring your right ankle up and place it on top of your left knee. Use your right hand to grab your right toes and gently pull them towards your ankle. Hold the position for two breaths and return foot to the starting position.
3. Repeat stretches on both feet two or three more times.

### Take Note:

- This stretch is helpful if you have plantar fasciitis or heel pain.
- If you cannot bring your ankle up to your knee, you can do this stretch by crossing your legs and stretching the foot by bringing your toes up towards your calf.

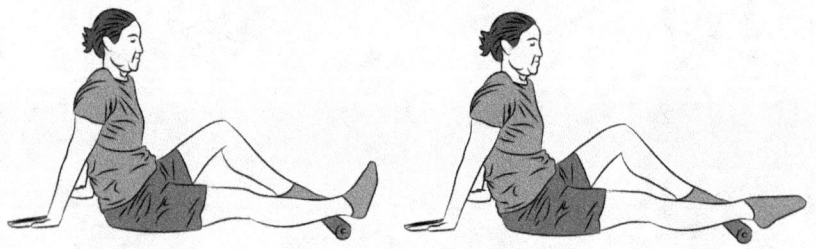

# Ankle Alphabet

**Areas Stretched: Ankles, Calves.**

1. Sit up straight on the floor with legs straight out in front of you. Your hands can be on the floor for support and balance.
2. Place a pillow or rolled up towel under your left calf so that your left foot and ankle are off the floor. Point your left foot and draw the letter A with your toes. Then draw the letter B, the letter C, and so forth. After you have completed the alphabet, switch the pillow to the other calf.
3. With your right calf supported by the pillow and right foot and ankle off the floor, point your right foot and draw the alphabet with your toes.

> **Take Note:**

- Don't worry if you find it hard to get through the entire alphabet the first few times. As you do this stretch regularly, your ankles will get stronger and your range of motion will increase.
- This stretch can also be done sitting in a chair.

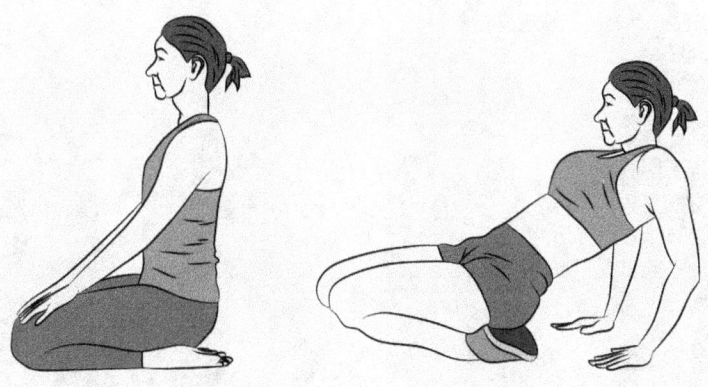

# Kneeling Shin Stretch

**Areas Stretched: Shins.**

1. Kneel on the floor or a padded mat, with your legs bent and feet behind you. Your knees should be touching each other. Slowly lower your buttocks and sit them down on the soles of your feet. Hold this position for two or three breaths in and out. Slowly come back up to the starting position.
2. Repeat the stretch two or three more times.

**Take Note:**

- Be sure your buttocks do not fall between your feet when you lower down. Keep your knees and feet together.
- If your knees do not allow you to sit all the way back onto your feet, come part way down or as far as you can. You may need to support yourself with hands on the floor or holding onto a sturdy chair.

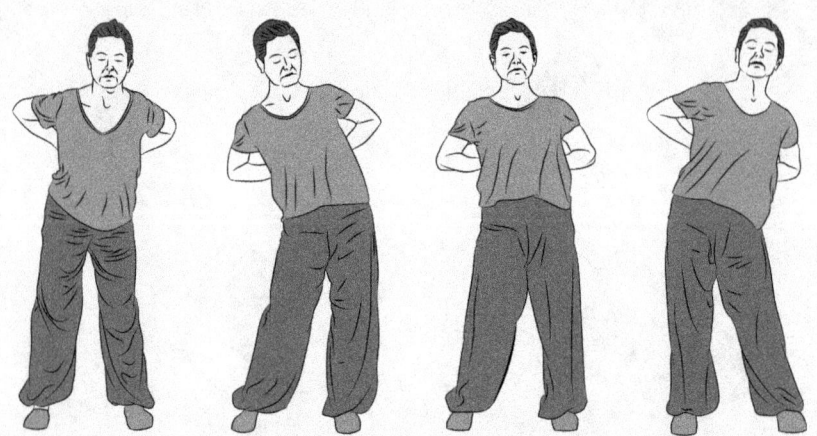

# Hip Rotations

### Areas Stretched: Hips.

1. Stand up tall with feet a little wider than hips width apart. Place your hands on your hips.
2. Keeping your feet firmly on the ground, move your hips clockwise in a large circle from one side, to the front, to the other side, and to the back. Make five large circles going in the same direction. Return to the starting position.
3. Now move your hips counterclockwise, going in the other direction, in a large circle. Make five large circles and then return to the starting position.
4. Repeat the hip rotations, going both ways, two or three more times.

### Take Note:

- Breathe normally while doing this stretch. Be sure that you are making large enough circles so that your hips are being stretched.
- Don't lock your knees but keep them slightly bent.

# Conclusion

Stretching is an important part of maintaining our body and general well-being as we progress into our later years of life. As we have learned throughout this book, stretching is for everyone, not just competitive athletes and professional dancers. A regular stretching routine can be done anywhere and at any time of the day. Stretching before and after exercise and strenuous activity is a no-brainer, but we saw that stretching in the morning and in the evening are not only beneficial but help us shift into and out of the events of our day.

There are many wrong ways to stretch that can actually hurt instead of help our bodies, so we learned some things to avoid. Remembering to first warm up before stretching is crucial as well as being careful to not bounce while stretching. Incorporating a variety of stretches is important to keep our muscles from any imbalances that may occur because of doing the same stretches again and again. The goal is muscle strength as well as symmetry. While we do want to stretch to the point of muscle tension, we have to stop before any stretch becomes painful because this is detrimental to our goal of flexibility and increased range of motion.

One of the goals in putting together this book of stretches was to provide a resource for older adults. Having a book that you can turn to again and again as you embark on a journey to better health through stretching is helpful. It is also convenient to have these stretches in one volume. The stretches in each chapter can be mixed and matched to fit your personal fitness goal and individual needs. As was mentioned previously, stretching is not a quick fix, but rather a lifestyle choice. Of the factors that contribute to our biological age, or the age at which our body functions, physical activity is one of the factors that we can easily control and easily pursue. While our chronological age, or how many years we have lived on this planet, can never change, our biological age can. The mobility and flexibility of our bodies help our biological age to always be younger than our natural born years.

All the best to you and to your health! If you enjoyed this book, please feel free to recommend it and leave a review on Amazon.

## Scan the QR code to leave a review:

I trust you will experience excellent health and well-being on the long road of life that lies before you and wish you my very best. Thank you for letting me share my knowledge with you.

Baz Thompson

# References

3 Easy Quad Stretches to Improve Thigh Flexibility. (2018). Verywell Fit. https://www.verywellfit.com/quadricep-stretches-2696366

American Council on Exercise. (2014, October 7). Top 10 Benefits of Stretching. Www.acefitness.org. https://www.acefitness.org/education-and-resources/lifestyle/blog/5107/top-10-benefits-of-stretching/

American Heart Association. (2014). Warm Up, Cool Down. Www.heart.org. https://www.heart.org/en/healthy-living/fitness/fitness-basics/warm-up-cool-down

Axtell, B. (2017, July 11). Foot Exercises: Strengthening, Flexibility, and More. Healthline. https://www.healthline.com/health/fitness-exercise/foot-exercises#toe-raise-point-and-curl

Batista, L. H., Vilar, A. C., de Almeida Ferreira, J. J., Rebelatto, J. R., & Salvini, T. F. (2009). Active stretching improves flexibility, joint torque, and functional mobility in older women. American Journal of Physical Medicine & Rehabilitation, 88(10), 815–822. https://doi.org/10.1097/PHM.0b013e3181b72149

Bumgardner, W. (2007, July 23). Shin Stretches for Your Anterior Tibialis. Verywell Fit; Verywell Fit. https://www.verywellfit.com/shin-stretches-standing-stetch-3436425

Cobra Abdominal Stretch / Old Horse Stretch – WorkoutLabs Exercise Guide. (n.d.). WorkoutLabs. Retrieved July 12, 2021, from https://workoutlabs.com/exercise-guide/cobra-abdominal-stretch/

Cronkleton, E. (2018, November 21). How to Get Rid of Lactic Acid in the Muscles. Healthline. https://www.healthline.com/health/how-to-get-rid-of-lactic-acid#warm-up

Cronkleton, E. (2019, July 12). Warmup Exercises: 6 Ways to Get Warmed Up Before a Workout. Healthline. https://www.healthline.com/health/fitness-exercise/warm-up-exercises#benefits

Davidson, K. (2021, April 20). Superman Exercise: How to Do It, Benefits, and Muscles Worked. Healthline. https://www.healthline.com/health/fitness/superman-exercise#muscles-worked

Eske, J. (2018, November 15). Best stretches for tight hamstrings: 7 methods. Www.medicalnewstoday.com. https://www.medicalnewstoday.com/articles/323703#7-best-hamstring-stretches

Evans, R. (2014, August 19). 4 Upper Back Stretches You Can Do at Your Desk. Healthline. https://www.healthline.com/health/back-pain/deskercize-upper-back#butterfly-wings

Gordon, D. (2021, January 28). 5 Ways to Perform Chest Stretches - wikiHow Fitness. Www.wikihow.fitness. https://www.wikihow.fitness/Perform-Chest-Stretches

Gudmestad, J. (2008, March 11). How to Stay Safe in Neck Rolls + Stretches | Yoga for your Neck. Yoga Journal. https://www.yogajournal.com/teach/how-to-stay-safe-in-neck-rolls-stretches/

Half Kneeling Hip Flexor Stretch | Functional Movement Systems. (n.d.). Www.functionalmovement.com. Retrieved July 7, 2021, from https://www.functionalmovement.com/Exercises/788/half_kneeling_hip_flexor_stretch

Harvard Health Publishing. (2013, September). The importance of stretching - Harvard Health. Harvard Health; Harvard Health. https://www.health.harvard.edu/staying-healthy/the-importance-of-stretching

Harvard Health Publishing. (2020, April 20). 5 exercises to improve hand mobility. Harvard Health. https://www.health.harvard.edu/pain/5-exercises-to-improve-hand-mobility

Higuera, V. (2020, November 23). Happy Baby Pose: How to Do, Benefits, and History. Healthline. https://www.healthline.com/health/happy-baby-pose

Hip Rotations. (n.d.). Www.workoutaholic.net. Retrieved July 13, 2021, from https://www.workoutaholic.net/exercises/hip_rotations

How to do Seated Spinal Twist. (n.d.). ClassPass. https://classpass.com/movements/seated-spinal-twist

How to do Thread the Needle Pose. (n.d.). ClassPass. Retrieved July 8, 2021, from https://classpass.com/movements/thread-the-needle-pose

Inverarity, L. (2005, November 23). Iliotibial (IT) Band Stretches to Treat ITBS. Verywell Fit; Verywell Fit. https://www.verywellfit.com/iliotibial-band-stretches-2696360

Lee, S. B., Oh, J. H., Park, J. H., Choi, S. P., & Wee, J. H. (2018). Differences in youngest-old, middle-old, and oldest-old patients who visit the emergency department. Clinical and Experimental Emergency Medicine, 5(4), 249–255. https://doi.org/10.15441/ceem.17.261

LoElizabeth. (2016, August 24). How To Yoga Fundamentals: Reclined Figure-4 To Prevent Injury. LoElizabeth Blog. http://loelizabeth.com/figure-4/

Lower Body Stretches. (n.d.). Www.arthritis.org. https://www.arthritis.org/health-wellness/healthy-living/physical-activity/success-strategies/lower-body-stretches

Marturana, A. (2019). 10 Great Stretches to Do After an Upper-Body Workout. SELF. https://www.self.com/gallery/upper-body-stretches

McCormick, R., & Vasilaki, A. (2018). Age-related changes in skeletal muscle: changes to life-style as a therapy. Biogerontology, 19(6), 519–536. https://doi.org/10.1007/s10522-018-9775-3

Meyler, Z. (2018, September 14). 4 Easy Stretches for a Stiff Neck. Spine-Health. https://www.spine-health.com/wellness/exercise/4-easy-stretches-stiff-neck

Miller, R. (2020, June 5). Easy Hamstring Stretches. Spine-Health. https://www.spine-health.com/wellness/exercise/easy-hamstring-stretches

National Center for Biotechnology Information, U.S. National Library of Medicine. (2020). What happens when you age? In www.ncbi.nlm.nih.gov. Institute for Quality and Efficiency in Health Care (IQWiG). https://www.ncbi.nlm.nih.gov/books/NBK563107/

Overhead Stretch. (n.d.). Www.exercise.com. https://www.exercise.com/exercises/overhead-stretch/

Pizer, A. (2021, May 24). How to Do Paschimottanasana, a Yoga Hamstring Stretch. Verywell Fit. https://www.verywellfit.com/seated-forward-bend-paschimottanasana-3567101

Posture of the Month: Banana Pose. (2018, October 5). Your Pace Yoga. https://yourpaceyoga.com/blog/posture-of-the-month-banana-pose/

Quinn, E. (2019a). The Basic Bridge Exercise for Core Stability. Verywell Fit. https://www.verywellfit.com/how-to-do-the-bridge-exercise-3120738

Quinn, E. (2019b, August 31). How to Do the Standing Lunge Stretch. Verywell Fit. https://www.verywellfit.com/performing-standing-lunge-stretch-3120306

Raye, J. (n.d.). Yin Yoga Square Pose with modifications. Jennifer Raye | Medicine and Movement. Retrieved July 12, 2021, from https://jenniferraye.com/blog/square-pose

Reclined Butterfly Pose. (n.d.). Ekhart Yoga. Retrieved July 8, 2021, from https://www.ekhartyoga.com/resources/yoga-poses/reclined-butterfly-pose

Schwengel, K. (2017, August 28). Lymph Flow Exercise: Floor Angels | Natural Balance Therapy. Naturalbalancetherapy.com. https://naturalbalancetherapy.com/self-treatment/lymph-flow-exercise-floor-angels/

Sleep Advisor. (2020, June 3). 8 Stretches for Your Best Night's Sleep. Sleep Advisor. https://www.sleepadvisor.org/stretching-before-bed/

Standing Twists / Trunk Rotations (Barbell) | Chunk Fitness. (2021). Chunkfitness.com. https://chunkfitness.com/exercises/ab-exercises/oblique-exercises/standing-twists-trunk-rotations-barbell

Stretch of the Week: Windshield Wiper Stretch. (2016, April 13). Athletico. https://www.athletico.com/2016/04/13/stretch-week-windshield-wiper-stretch/

Stretch22. (n.d.). The Top Benefits of Stretching in the Morning. Stretch 22. Retrieved July 7, 2021, from https://stretch22.com/wake-and-stretch-the-top-benefits-of-stretching-in-the-morning/

Sugar, J. (2018, December 23). This Is Our Favorite Stretch to Do in Bed: Cat and Cow. POPSUGAR Fitness. https://www.popsugar.com/fitness/Relieve-Back-Pain-Cat-Cow-Stretch-8320711

Supine Spinal Twist Can Help Improve Back Mobility. (n.d.). Verywell Fit. Retrieved July 8, 2021, from https://www.verywellfit.com/supine-spinal-twist-supta-matsyendrasana-3567125

Tight Shoulders: 12 Stretches for Fast Relief and Tips for Prevention. (2018, January 12). Healthline. https://www.healthline.com/health/tight-shoulders#stretches

Top 10 shoulder stretches for pain and tightness. (2019, March 8). Www.medicalnewstoday.com. https://www.medicalnewstoday.com/articles/324647#shoulder-rolls

Tucker, A. (2018). 5 Essential Calf Stretches Everyone Should Be Doing. SELF. https://www.self.com/gallery/essential-calf-stretches

Volpi, E., Nazemi, R., & Fujita, S. (2004). Muscle tissue changes with aging. Current Opinion in Clinical Nutrition and Metabolic Care, 7(4), 405–410. https://doi.org/10.1097/01.mco.0000134362.76653.b2

Walker, B. (2010, August 27). What is stretching? How to stretch properly? When to stretch? Stretch Coach. https://stretchcoach.com/articles/how-to-stretch/

Yoga Poses Dictionary | Pocket Yoga. (n.d.). Www.pocketyoga.com. Retrieved July 6, 2021, from https://www.pocketyoga.com/pose/mountain_cactus_arms

www.ingramcontent.com/pod-product-compliance
Lightning Source LLC
Chambersburg PA
CBHW081311070526
44578CB00006B/837